Drug Discovery: Innovations in
the 21st Century

Drug Discovery: Innovations in the 21st Century

Editor: Ned Burnett

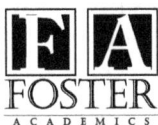

FA

FOSTER
ACADEMICS

www.fosteracademics.com

www.fosteracademics.com

FA
FOSTER
ACADEMICS

Cataloging-in-Publication Data

Drug discovery : innovations in the 21st century / edited by Ned Burnett.
    p. cm.
Includes bibliographical references and index.
ISBN 978-1-63242-586-7
1. Drugs. 2. Drug development--History--21st century.
3. Pharmaceutical technology. I. Burnett, Ned.
RS91 .D78 2019
615.1--dc23

© Foster Academics, 2019

Foster Academics,
118-35 Queens Blvd., Suite 400,
Forest Hills, NY 11375, USA

ISBN 978-1-63242-586-7 (Hardback)

Contents

Permissions

List of Contributors

Index

Contents

Preface

The main aim of this book is to educate learners and enhance their research focus by presenting diverse topics covering this vast field. This is an advanced book which compiles significant studies by distinguished experts in the area of analysis. This book addresses successive solutions to the challenges arising in the area of application, along with it; the book provides scope for future developments.

Drugs are usually derived from natural sources, such as plant derived natural products, microbial metabolites, marine invertebrate derived compounds, etc. Drug discovery is an interdisciplinary field of medicine, pharmacology and biotechnology, which is concerned with the process of discovery of potential new medications. Modern drug discovery is a complex process, which involves a number of technical procedures such as identification of screening hits and their optimization to increase the selectivity, potency, affinity, metabolic stability and oral bioavailability of the hits. When a compound fulfills all of these requirements, it proceeds towards drug development and clinical trials. This book elucidates the concepts and innovative models around prospective developments with respect to drug discovery. It provides significant information of this domain to help develop a good understanding of drug discovery and related fields. With state-of-the-art inputs by acclaimed experts of this field, this book targets students and professionals.

It was a great honour to edit this book, though there were challenges, as it involved a lot of communication and networking between me and the editorial team. However, the end result was this all-inclusive book covering diverse themes in the field.

Finally, it is important to acknowledge the efforts of the contributors for their excellent chapters, through which a wide variety of issues have been addressed. I would also like to thank my colleagues for their valuable feedback during the making of this book.

Editor

Going Small: Using Biophysical Screening to Implement Fragment Based Drug Discovery

John J. Bowling, William R. Shadrick,

Elizabeth C. Griffith and Richard E. Lee

Additional information is available at the end of the chapter

Abstract

Screening against biochemical targets with compact chemical fragments has developed a reputation as a successful early-stage drug discovery approach, thanks to recent drug approvals. Having weak initial target affinities, fragments require the use of sensitive biophysical technologies (NMR, SPR, thermal shift, ITC, and X-ray crystallography) to accommodate the practical limits of going smaller. Application of optimized fragment biophysical screening approaches now routinely allows for the rapid identification of fragments with high binding efficiencies. The aim of this chapter is to provide an introduction to fragment library selection and to discuss the suitability of screening approaches adapted for lower-throughput biophysical techniques. A general description of metrics that are being used in the progression of fragment hits, the need for orthogonal assay testing, and guidance on potential pitfalls are included to assist scientists, considering initiating their own fragment discovery program.

Keywords: fragment-based drug discovery, biophysical screening, efficiency metrics, nuclear magnetic resonance spectroscopy, surface plasmon resonance, thermal shift assay, isothermal titration calorimetry, fluorescence polarization, X-ray crystallography

1. Introduction

"Going small" with fragment-based drug discovery (FBDD) denotes using low molecular weight compounds to probe a therapeutic target. This also includes using smaller tailored libraries and lower screening throughput in more carefully measured assays. This is a consequence of being reliant on biophysical technologies, as compared to classical high-throughput screening (HTS) approaches performed in 384-well plates that detect product formation. FBDD at its core is target-based drug discovery, but the initial approach of fragment screening differs from standard lead-like screening, which utilizes much larger higher molecular weight screening libraries.

In theory, modern target-based drug discovery screening libraries are designed to maximize coverage of chemical space. This is especially important for groups that use high-throughput technologies (HTS) and screen against diverse targets. These target-based programs tend to rely on screening the highest practical number of chemical entities from their screening libraries, sometimes accumulating millions of compounds [1]. However, with over 166 billion possible synthetically accessible organic molecules containing up to 17 heavy atoms (nonhydrogen) [2], even the biggest screening libraries cannot possibly statistically represent this vast chemical space [3].

From modeling described in a 2001 article, Hann and colleagues showed how higher molecular complexity (i.e., ligand size) significantly decreased the probability of protein-site molecular recognition [4]. The authors outlined this as a primary shortcoming of the combinatorial chemistry/HTS approach to drug discovery and promoted the idea that screening smaller libraries with reduced complexity could be a complementary approach. Thus, by reducing compound complexity, FBDD evades the pitfall of scaffold bias which develops in large lead-like screening libraries.

In this chapter, the reader should come to appreciate how going small is an intrinsically orthogonal screening platform that is easily integrated with established biophysical techniques. The methods, examples, and citations discussed are intended to guide a newcomer to FBDD, specifically scientists who have some prior experience with drug screening principles.

2. The rise of fragments as a screening ideology

Fragment-based drug discovery started as a concept published in 1981 [5] by biochemist William P. Jencks, who characterized the binding affinities of molecules to proteins as being built from components. Citing several examples, he described how the balance of Gibbs-free energy for a two-component molecule binding to a protein could also be described through the equation $\Delta G^0_{AB} = \Delta G^i_A + \Delta G^i_B + \Delta G^s$, where ΔG^i values are the "intrinsic binding energies" of the components and ΔG^s is their "connection Gibbs energy." A key aspect of the concept is that the component's contribution to the balance of the observed binding energy (ΔG^0_{AB}) would be relatively significant but weak, thus creating a challenge for detection. Jencks' concept was obscured at the time due to the excitement around combi-chem/HTS drug discovery approaches. In 1996, the conceptual observations of Jencks were experimentally validated by the team of Fesik. His team successfully produced a drug lead by linking fragment hits detected by a sensitive two-dimensional nuclear magnetic resonance (NMR) spectroscopy binding assay (often referred to as SAR-by-NMR) [6]. Since then, fragment-based drug discovery has energized the pharmaceutical industry. In 2011, a drug for BRAF-mutated metastatic melanoma became the first FDA-approved drug discovered via FBDD [7]. A second, for chronic lymphocytic leukemia, was approved in 2016 [8], with several related candidates currently making their way through the pipeline [9].

3. Fragment primary screening

At present, NMR, surface plasmon resonance (SPR), thermal shift assay (TSA), isothermal titration calorimetry (ITC), and X-ray crystallography (Sections 3.2–3.4, 4.1 and 4.2) are the most widely used techniques in FDBB. Given their respective throughput capacities NMR, SPR, and TSA are often used as the primary screening technology with ITC and X-ray crystallography reserved as secondary screening. **Figure 1** shows the effective ligand affinity coverage of each technique which partly demonstrates their utility with FBDD. All biophysical screening techniques work best in combination and individual hits need careful orthogonal validation. Crystallography is the gold standard as the information gained allows for rapid ligand advancement. However, its application as a primary screen is often impractical due to resource and time limitations. High concentration inhibitor biochemical or fluorescence polarization (FP) assays can be used in some cases for orthogonal validation of primary screening hits where crystallography is not an option.

The workflow represented in **Figure 2** shows how these techniques might be organized into a traditional screening paradigm. It is common to use some of these techniques in parallel, particularly at the secondary screening stage since there are always fewer compounds to evaluate. Pragmatically, scientists should obtain structural insights at this secondary stage to validate primary screening results. Structural information is preferred when deciding to progress a fragment to the hit generation stage (discussed further in Section 5.2).

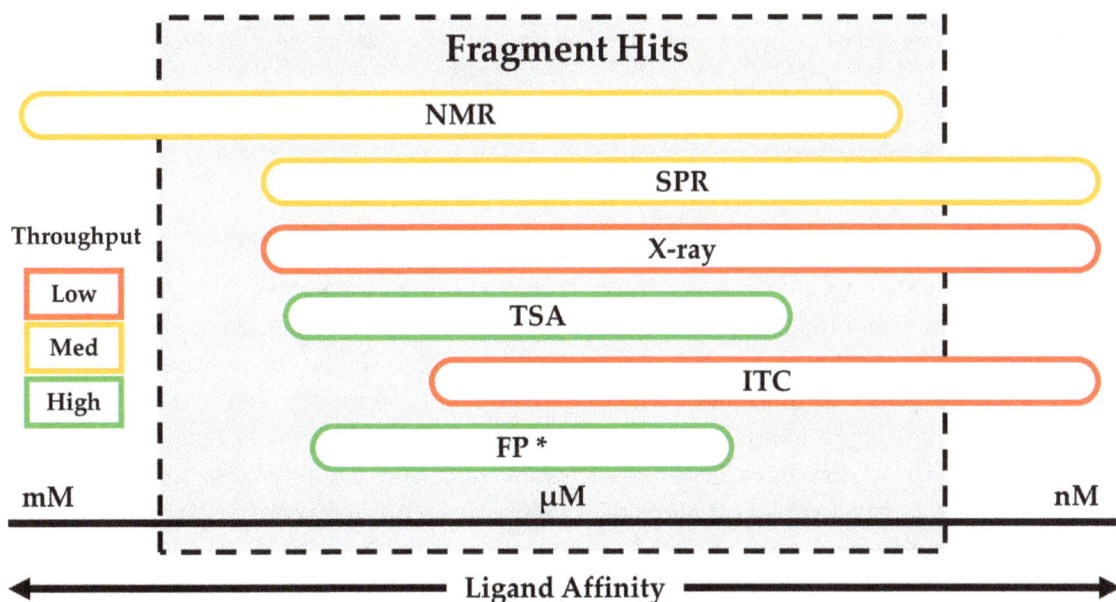

Figure 1. The range of fragment affinities covered by the biophysical techniques described in this chapter. The techniques are ranked from the top downwards in order of their typical frequency of use in FBDD programs (SPR being a close second). NMR (yellow outline) is represented as a medium-throughput method but can be low-throughput based on the availability of protein and whether recycling is required. *Fluorescence polarization, technically a biochemical technique and highly dependent on probe affinity, is included for comparison but can be applied to fragment screening.

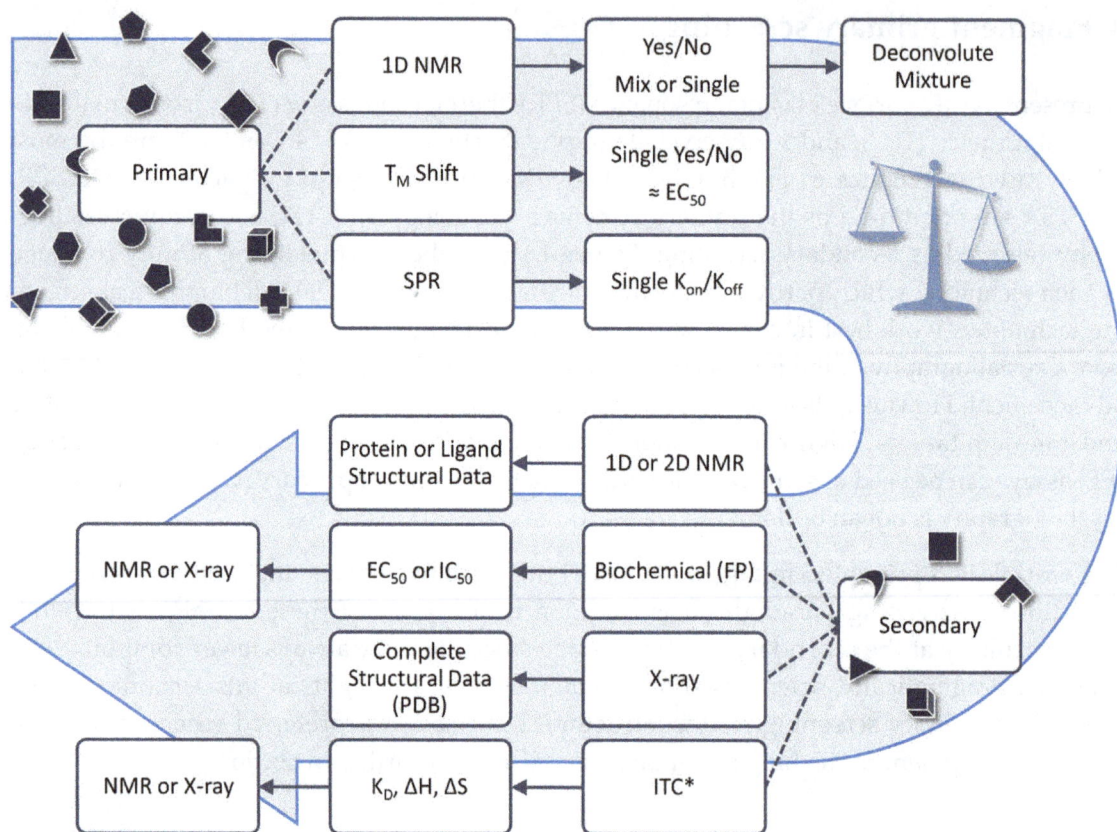

Figure 2. An example of the typical FBDD screening workflow. The workflow assumes structural information by X-ray or NMR. The hierarchy will not accurately depict the resources of all drug discovery programs. Dashed connections represent screening options at the primary and secondary screening stages. Arrows point to the results from each screen to be ranked or compared to those of other techniques. Fragments promoted to secondary screening will eventually require structural information to be progressed to hit generation. *The ITC technique is typically used for ranking fragment hits after secondary screening.

3.1. Fragment library design

An obvious first step for any primary fragment screening is to resource compounds for the screen. However, wielding a proper fragment library as a tool for hit generation conflicts with traditional lead-like screening methods. Central to the conflict is the regular use of high concentrations of compounds to accommodate expected low binding affinities. Practical pitfalls, such as compound aggregation, compound precipitation, dramatic pH changes, detector saturation, and nonspecific interactions, are a minor concern when nanomolar concentrations are used during screening of larger molecular weight molecules, but can become major issues when millimolar concentrations are used in fragment screening.

In 2003, scientists at Astex Pharmaceuticals published a synopsis of their emerging fragment drug-discovery program and noted that the average physical properties of their fragment hits fell conveniently within different orders of 3 (molecular weight <300, hydrogen bond donors ≤3, hydrogen bond acceptors ≤3, and ClogP ≤3) [10]. As a compliment to Lipinski's rule of 5 (RO5), the fragment rule of 3 (RO3) was a convenient target toward which chemical suppliers built fragment libraries from their existing stores. Ten years later, Astex Pharmaceuticals revised their position [11], stating that similar to the RO5 described by Lipinski, RO3 was more of a guideline and that their refined library consisted of fragments with less than 17 heteroatoms with molecular mass <230 Daltons. This exemplifies how well-constructed fragment libraries should rely heavily on practicality to be effective tools and speaks to the need for additional scrutiny of (in order of importance) solubility, stability, and reactivity for effective fragment screening.

Commercial and nonprofit access to fragment libraries exists, and several examples have been characterized [12, 13]. A custom library allows for existing libraries to be used in addition to catalog resources with some tailoring based on specific cheminformatics principles, such as optimization of the representative chemical space, avoidance of nuisance compounds, and guidance with pharmacophore models. One early stage example of note is the Global Fragment Initiative (GFI) by Pfizer [14], wherein the library was built from compounds on hand, purchased, and synthesized. Each member of the GFI library was rigorously characterized and empirically tested for aqueous solubility up to 1 mM, with the intent of using the library for multiple biophysical techniques. How a fragment library is procured will depend on an acceptable balance of convenience and cost, but it is highly recommended that the end user have methods in place to reliably assess each compound for practical use at high concentrations. For an example of this workflow, see **Figure 3**.

Fragment hits can have limited traction toward chemical expansion or linking as a consequence of their size. As a safeguard, Merck strategically redesigned its general FBDD library to accommodate more structure-activity relationships and to fill structural gaps by visual inspection [15]. The purposeful move away from diversity in its general library was a concerted effort of cheminformatics and crowdsourcing of medicinal chemists to gain pipeline traction. The strategy leads to larger general screening libraries and effectively restricts widespread application to appropriately equipped programs. Regardless, any FBDD program

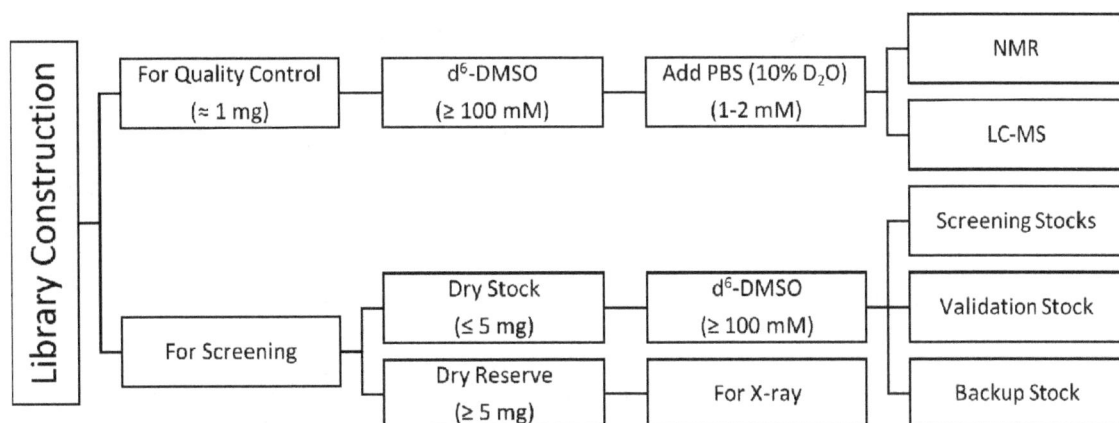

Figure 3. A suggested library construction workflow for FBDD. Once compounds are obtained as dry stocks, the workflow proceeds left to right. Having redundancy built into the screening stocks helps rule out contamination or mishandling. It is presumed that fragments will eventually be used in NMR studies, therefore dissolved using deuterated solvents (d6-DMSO and D$_2$O). Rigid quality control is recommended to eliminate spoiled or misidentified compounds and repeated on hits or on the event of significant additions of fragments to the library.

design must account for this pitfall and ensure the potential to develop fragment hits through chemistry or catalogs.

Finally, Pan-Assay Interference Compounds (PAINS) are a well-known classification of chemical entities to activity across multiple assays and proteins, and they have been thoroughly reviewed in regards to their practical impacts on FBDD [16], and related cheminformatics filters are available via the Internet [17]. The reduced chemical complexity of fragments does inherently diminish the number of "worst offenders" in its library and often bad fragments are quickly identified and triaged from screening libraries.

In conclusion, for FBDD, it is prudent to prioritize highly soluble fragment libraries with a diversity of ring shapes that can match a broad range of hydrogen bonding interactions from the protein target. A minimalistic approach would be to only eliminate mostly predictable fragment "show stoppers," containing toxicophores subject to xenobiotic metabolism, since it is often easy to scaffold hop in the early stages of FBDD to remove unwanted motifs.

3.2. Nuclear magnetic resonance

Modern NMR spectroscopy is best known for enabling the three-dimensional characterization of ordered molecular structures in solution and was the first technique to be used for fragment screening [6]. It is also one of the few biophysical techniques that can easily be switched between perspectives of the small molecule and the protein at run time. A growing list of NMR experiments used in fragment screening can help validate hits without using additional biophysical techniques.

Samples are prepared *in situ* by using automation (such as the Gilson GX-271 in **Figure 4**) or by pipetting manually. One immediate benefit of the manual method is the ease with which a scientist can eliminate precipitated or turbid samples by optical analytics. Individual inspection of samples is time-consuming but a must for any successful FBDD program, providing important feedback about the fragment library. Fragments must be dissolved in deuterated solvent (e.g., 99.9% d6-DMSO, Cambridge Isotope Laboratories, Inc., USA) for programs using NMR at any stage (see **Figure 3**). Typical concentration ratios for test samples are 10:1 up to 30:1 fragment to protein in the chosen buffer (phosphate buffers being the most common). Prior knowledge of the K_d and stoichiometry is not required but can be used to tune concentrations to avoid unintended site saturation by an individual fragment, which is a general concern when screening fragment mixtures or performing competition experiments. Finally, the issue of whether or not to use surfactants (e.g., 0.05% Triton X100) to help eliminate false positives is best left to a case by case basis, but if used, the conditions should be consistent with orthogonal techniques, with the exception of crystallography.

Spectroscopy experiments that indicate binding from the fragment's perspective are structurally less informative but have a higher dynamic range than do protein-detected experiments. Because significant cost savings can be made by using unlabeled protein, early-stage, budget-conscious programs may focus on using the ligand-detected suite of experiments shown in **Figure 4**, often acquiring them in parallel for each sample. The saturation transfer difference (STD) experiment can provide a binding-epitope map, as magnetization can only travel

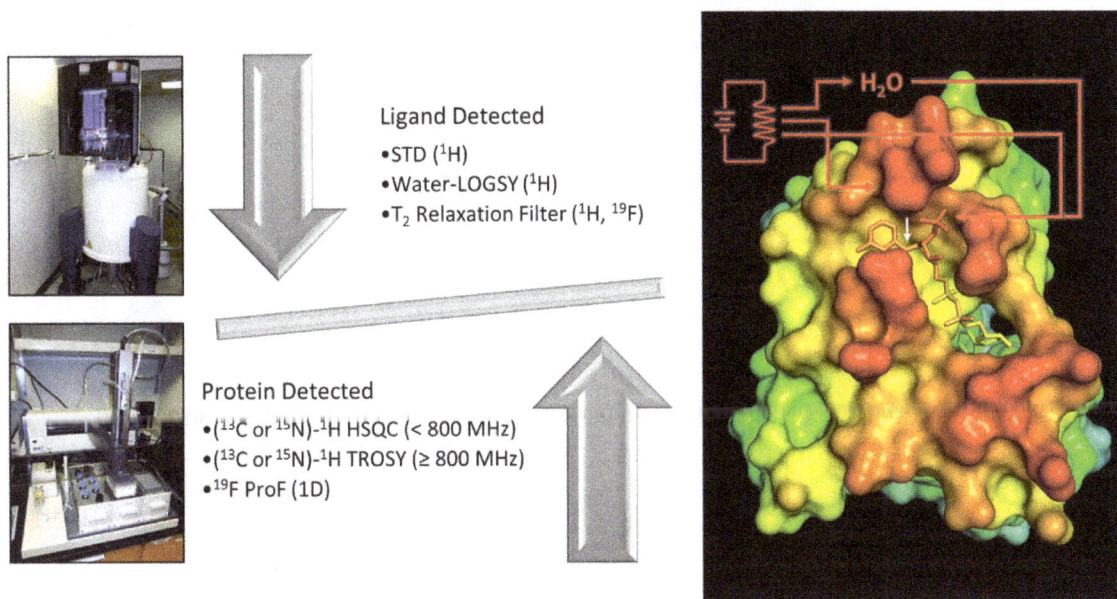

Figure 4. Screening fragments by NMR may include the use of automated sample preparation and handling. Common NMR experiments used in FBDD programs are listed, categorized according to their use of the magnetization pathways indicated. For ligand-detected experiments, additional pathways to the unbound ligand also exist. The white arrow indicates magnetization transfer from the protein to its bound ligand and is specific to the saturation transfer difference (STD) experiment.

through the protein to the bound fragment [18]. The epitope map enables a scientist using unlabeled protein to identify the portions of the fragment in closest proximity to the protein and, conversely, the portions available for expansion or linking for hit generation. Specialized experiments, such as the interligand nuclear Overhauser effect and target immobilized NMR screening (ILOE [19] and TINS [20], respectively), are best reserved for the study of difficult proteins or competition experiments. From the protein perspective, several variants of the two-dimensional HSQC experiment (typically ^{1}H nuclei measured directly and X nuclei, indirectly) that helps to disperse the numerous signals in a protein target and depend on the protein isotopic enrichment strategy. TROSY (another HSQC variant) can be used for large, usually perdeuterated proteins but requires a high-field instrument (i.e., 800 MHz and up); the discovery of methods to selectively label methyls [21] has simplified the resulting spectra and enabled screening on lower-field instruments (e.g., 500 MHz) [22].

To reduce protein consumption, NMR FBDD relies on the screening of equimolar fragment mixtures. This step is immediately followed by mixture dereplication, usually involving manual interpretation of spectra, although with careful sample preparation and a well-curated fragment spectral database, hits can be identified by software (e.g., *Mnova Suite*, Mestrelab Research S.L.; *ACD/Spectrus Suite*, Advanced Chemistry Development, Inc.; *Topspin*, Bruker Inc.). Individual reference spectra are acquired during the quality control steps of the fragment library design, and mixtures are then designed to avoid spectral overlap and reactivity. The number of fragments used per mixture is not standardized; but, basic statistical principles support using as few fragments as possible while avoiding mixing acids with bases or nucleophiles with electrophiles. For ^{1}H-observed experiments, 5–7 compounds per mixture is a reasonable starting point. Validation of hits is accomplished by a second round of screening individual fragments. At the validation stage, the use of spectroscopy experiments that provide binding site information (e.g., HSQC, STD mapping, ILOE) is highly recommended if crystallography is not readily available. Any resulting structural information is crucial for promoting the fragment into the downstream processes of medicinal chemistry and hit generation.

With the exception of WaterLOGSY, titration and analysis of the resulting signal of these NMR experiments can provide binding affinity scores for fragments with reasonable accuracy. In addition to the previously described STD experiment, ^{19}F NMR screening by filtered transverse relaxation (T_2), a filter also referred to as a Carr-Purcell-Meiboom-Gill (CPMG) scheme, can be a powerful option if used in competition with a known fluorinated ligand having a K_d measured carefully by using more rigorous techniques (e.g., SPR, ITC, FP). The potential benefit is that one sample can be analyzed for fragments in competition with or, perhaps, having an allosteric contribution to binding, and binding affinity is back-calculated relative to an internal nonbinding control or electric reference signal [23].

There are relatively few drawbacks to using available NMR facilities in a FBDD program considering the method's ability to contribute to every aspect of the workflow, such as library quality control and hit generation. The two drawbacks that are most often cited are the speed of the screen from sample preparation to data analysis and the demands on protein production for screening by NMR.

3.3. Surface plasmon resonance

Surface plasmon resonance shares the spotlight with NMR as a major screening technique for FBDD programs. The hurdles that come with using an immobilized protein for screening are counterbalanced by increased sensitivity and immediate access to kinetics data. Although absolute binding kinetics are not assured when dealing with weak affinities, for well-optimized experiments, obtaining k_a (binding), k_d (dissociation) rates, and the K_D (binding constant) value is certainly possible. Consequently, interpreting the resulting sensorgram can be challenging; but thankfully, the biosensor community has over 25 years of experiments to help set standards—hundreds just in 2009 [24]. With improvements in software to include experiment wizards, relatively new users can screen numerous fragments.

These experiments generally have long lead in times, as protein immobilization chemistry and buffer conditions need to be carefully perfected prior to screening experiments. Setting aside the routine instrument maintenance and screen validation using appropriate controls, the traditional stages of each experiment have been buffer and compound preparation, target immobilization, start-up samples (i.e., buffer match, blanks, and positive controls), fragment primary screen, data reduction and analysis, hit selection, and secondary dose response of hits.

Successful FBDD programs focus most practical attention on the preparation of the chip immobilization surface, ensuring stability between experiments. This focus on stability assumes that the loading conditions for the protein have been standardized and validated across multiple coupling methods, such as a covalent amine coupling [25] (to amine termini or lysine) or the less-amenable (regarding FBDD) coupling by protein tags (e.g., biotinylation or poly-histidine).

Once the target is loaded, screening samples should be prepared as single-point concentrations, for example 100 µM. The concentrations can be variable, but the expectation is that they are carefully prepared to avoid common problems such as precipitation and aggregate formation that may produce nonstoichiometric binding to the target. The use of detergents is allowable for the sake of the target but further complicates buffer matching in the reference channel. Troublesome fragments identified by their atypical sensorgrams are usually triaged from screening collections.

Once the data have been collected, data reduction and normalization follows and requires some practice to prosecute these steps efficiently. An experienced scientist can perform a first pass of the entire data set to quickly exclude sensorgrams for which a reasonable curve fit is unlikely due to compound incompatibilities or systemic problems with the instrument (**Figure 5**). Next, data reduction can seem like a tedious process to simply "clean" the sensorgrams; but in addition to aligning the injection time points, it checks the soundness of the blank injections, which yield important problem-solving data. Finally, the configuration of most instruments requires multiple runs to cover entire fragment libraries, so run-to-run variation naturally exists. Normalization seeks to enable the comparison of experimental responses, regardless of target density, binding activity, molecular weight, and buffer mismatch. The most expedient way to achieve this is by using the known concentration and bind-

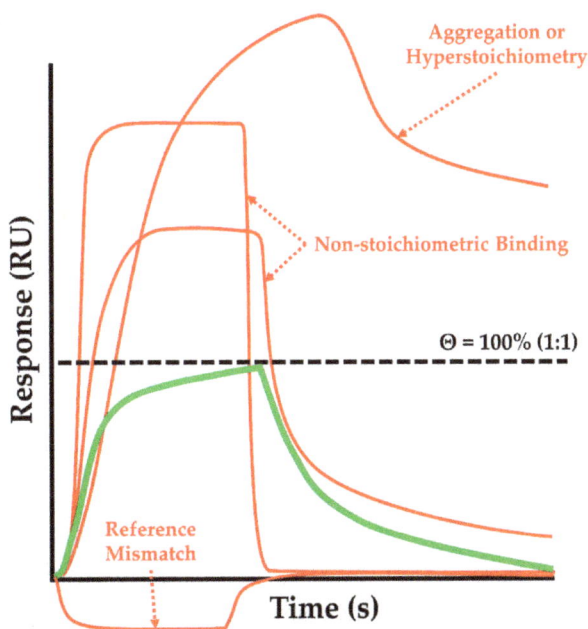

Figure 5. Ideal (green) and unfortunate (red) sensorgrams simulate binding and nonbinding events during the SPR experiment. Aggregation is typically concentration-dependent, whereas incorrect stoichiometry will not fit simple binding models. Relative occupancy (θ) of 100%, with a 1:1 stoichiometry indicated at the dashed line, represents how using high concentrations of fragments that appear to bind do so nonspecifically, binding weakly to multiple sites on the protein, chip surface, or nothing at all.

ing affinities of the control compound injections to convert the response unit (RU) to a relative occupancy (θ), wherein 100% would be saturated binding (i.e., R_{eq}/R_{max}).

Recently developed methods have increased the throughput of dose response studies, providing kinetic information earlier in the screening workflow and practically eliminating the need for a secondary set of experiments for hits. For example, a nonbinding diluent (i.e., 20%, w/v sucrose) can be used to create a range of compound concentrations from the same sample [26], or individually prepared sample concentrations can be sequentially injected (e.g., "single cycle kinetics" or kinetic titration) [27]. Both methods save time by avoiding multiple regeneration steps. Further gains have been realized by using Taylor dispersion injections [28] in a longer flow path (e.g., OneStep™, SensiQ Technologies Inc.) to deliberately produce a gradient of analyte concentration flowing across the chip surface: by modeling [29] this dispersion from a known initial concentration, the same kinetic data can be obtained during the injection phase of the experiment.

3.4. Thermal shift assay

Protein exists in a thermodynamic equilibrium between the folded and unfolded state. As the temperature of the system increases, the ratio of folded to unfolded protein shifts toward the unfolded state, making it possible to determine the temperature at which half of the protein is in the unfolded state. This point is referred to as the melting temperature of the protein (T_m). The thermal shift assay relies on ligand-induced conformational stabilization, which is based on the energetic coupling of ligand binding and protein denaturation. In short, fragment binding alters the ratio of folded to unfolded protein by stabilizing the folded state (**Figure 6**). Adding a stabilizing fragment will shift the T_m, allowing for the calculation of ΔT_m

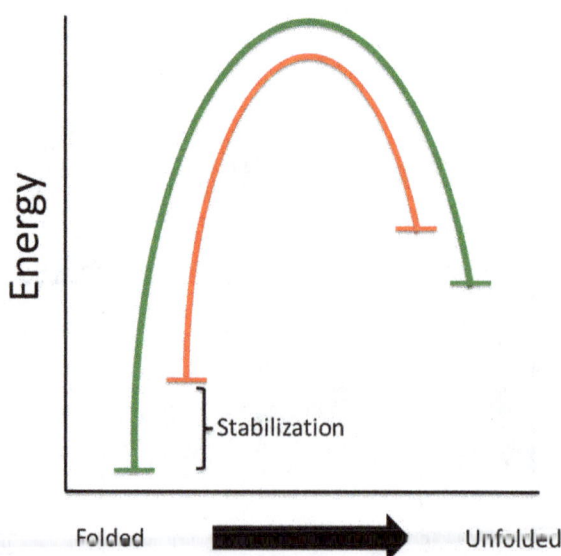

Figure 6. This figure demonstrates the theory associated with thermal shift interactions. Ligand binding causes stabilization of the protein in the more ordered folded state (represented in green). Thus, more thermal energy is required to move ligand stabilized protein from the folded to the unfolded state. Protein in the absence of ligand is represented in red. This protein requires less thermal energy to shift to the disordered state.

or lysine) or the less-amenable (regarding FBDD) coupling by protein tags (e.g., biotinylation or poly-histidine).

Once the target is loaded, screening samples should be prepared as single-point concentrations, for example 100 μM. The concentrations can be variable, but the expectation is that they are carefully prepared to avoid common problems such as precipitation and aggregate formation that may produce nonstoichiometric binding to the target. The use of detergents is allowable for the sake of the target but further complicates buffer matching in the reference channel. Troublesome fragments identified by their atypical sensorgrams are usually triaged from screening collections.

Once the data have been collected, data reduction and normalization follows and requires some practice to prosecute these steps efficiently. An experienced scientist can perform a first pass of the entire data set to quickly exclude sensorgrams for which a reasonable curve fit is unlikely due to compound incompatibilities or systemic problems with the instrument (**Figure 5**). Next, data reduction can seem like a tedious process to simply "clean" the sensorgrams; but in addition to aligning the injection time points, it checks the soundness of the blank injections, which yield important problem-solving data. Finally, the configuration of most instruments requires multiple runs to cover entire fragment libraries, so run-to-run variation naturally exists. Normalization seeks to enable the comparison of experimental responses, regardless of target density, binding activity, molecular weight, and buffer mismatch. The most expedient way to achieve this is by using the known concentration and bind-

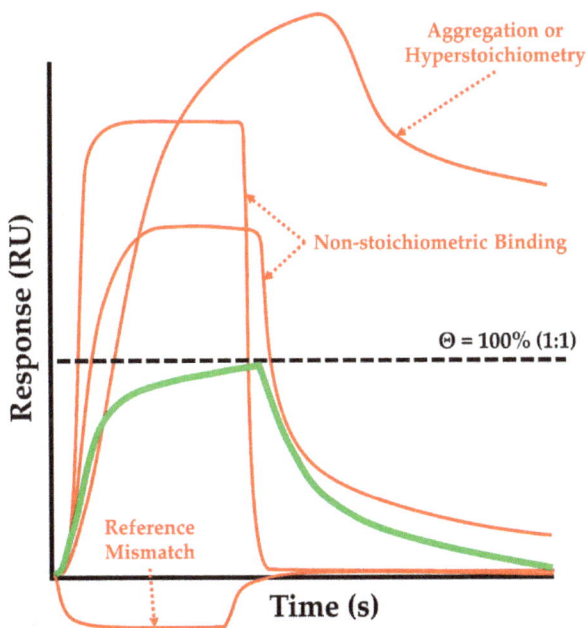

Figure 5. Ideal (green) and unfortunate (red) sensorgrams simulate binding and nonbinding events during the SPR experiment. Aggregation is typically concentration-dependent, whereas incorrect stoichiometry will not fit simple binding models. Relative occupancy (θ) of 100%, with a 1:1 stoichiometry indicated at the dashed line, represents how using high concentrations of fragments that appear to bind do so nonspecifically, binding weakly to multiple sites on the protein, chip surface, or nothing at all.

ing affinities of the control compound injections to convert the response unit (RU) to a relative occupancy (θ), wherein 100% would be saturated binding (i.e., R_{eq}/R_{max}).

Recently developed methods have increased the throughput of dose response studies, providing kinetic information earlier in the screening workflow and practically eliminating the need for a secondary set of experiments for hits. For example, a nonbinding diluent (i.e., 20%, w/v sucrose) can be used to create a range of compound concentrations from the same sample [26], or individually prepared sample concentrations can be sequentially injected (e.g., "single cycle kinetics" or kinetic titration) [27]. Both methods save time by avoiding multiple regeneration steps. Further gains have been realized by using Taylor dispersion injections [28] in a longer flow path (e.g., OneStep™, SensiQ Technologies Inc.) to deliberately produce a gradient of analyte concentration flowing across the chip surface: by modeling [29] this dispersion from a known initial concentration, the same kinetic data can be obtained during the injection phase of the experiment.

3.4. Thermal shift assay

Protein exists in a thermodynamic equilibrium between the folded and unfolded state. As the temperature of the system increases, the ratio of folded to unfolded protein shifts toward the unfolded state, making it possible to determine the temperature at which half of the protein is in the unfolded state. This point is referred to as the melting temperature of the protein (T_m). The thermal shift assay relies on ligand-induced conformational stabilization, which is based on the energetic coupling of ligand binding and protein denaturation. In short, fragment binding alters the ratio of folded to unfolded protein by stabilizing the folded state (**Figure 6**). Adding a stabilizing fragment will shift the T_m, allowing for the calculation of ΔT_m

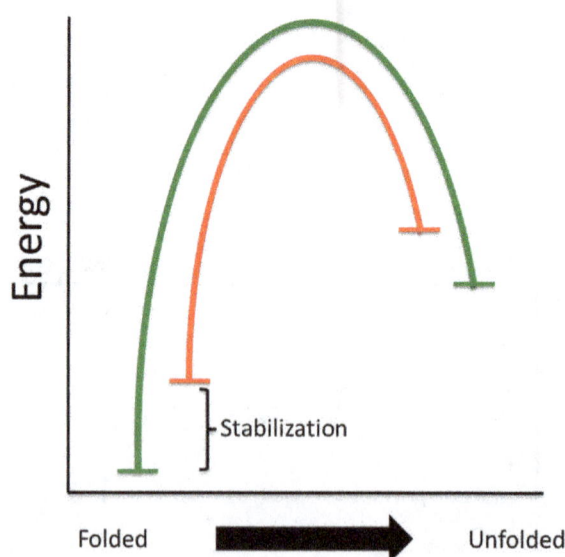

Figure 6. This figure demonstrates the theory associated with thermal shift interactions. Ligand binding causes stabilization of the protein in the more ordered folded state (represented in green). Thus, more thermal energy is required to move ligand stabilized protein from the folded to the unfolded state. Protein in the absence of ligand is represented in red. This protein requires less thermal energy to shift to the disordered state.

as an indicator of fragment binding [30–32]. Several methods available to measure the ratio of folded to unfolded protein in a given condition are: circular dichroism, infrared spectroscopy, differential scanning calorimetry, measurement of the intrinsic fluorescence of exposed tryptophan residues, and TSA, which is the most commonly applied technique. These methods were first adapted for use in TSA as a simple and inexpensive biophysical method for drug discovery in 2001 [30]. This work determined that ligand-induced protein stabilization could be tracked with environmentally sensitive dyes over a range of experimental temperatures. In an aqueous environment, the dye is quenched, giving minimal quantum yield. As the protein is denatured in the increasing temperature, its hydrophobic core is exposed to react with the dye. This interaction measurably increases the quantum yield of the dye.

Thermal shift has since been revised and optimized for use as an economical fragment screening method. A typical TSA has minimal requirements for the quantity of the target protein. A pilot assay should be completed wherein the concentration of protein is altered over a given range, as running TSA with an excess of protein can saturate the detector. Alternatively, too little protein will give a flat curve and negatively affect the signal-to-noise ratio in the resulting data (**Figure 7**). Thermal shift assays are commonly completed with 1–10 μM target protein, which should be as pure as possible. Gross impurities within the sample protein could lead to multiple curves, reducing the accuracy of the resulting data.

In addition to protein, TSA requires an environmentally sensitive dye. Historically napthylamine sulfonic acid dyes (such as 1,8-ANS, 2,6-ANS, or 2,6-TNS) were used for this purpose. Currently, SYPRO Orange is used more commonly as its fluorescence (Ex/Em of 300, 550/630 nm) is better adapted to rtPCR instruments. This dye is supplied from the vendor as a 5000X concentrate in DMSO. A pilot assay should be conducted to determine the appropriate concentration of SYPRO Orange for a given assay, as is done for protein concentration. In practice, many assays can be effectively run at a 5X concentration of SYPRO Orange. After the appropriate dye concentration has been established, a master mix of dye and buffer can be applied to the assay plate. At this point the plate is ready for the application of a fragment library.

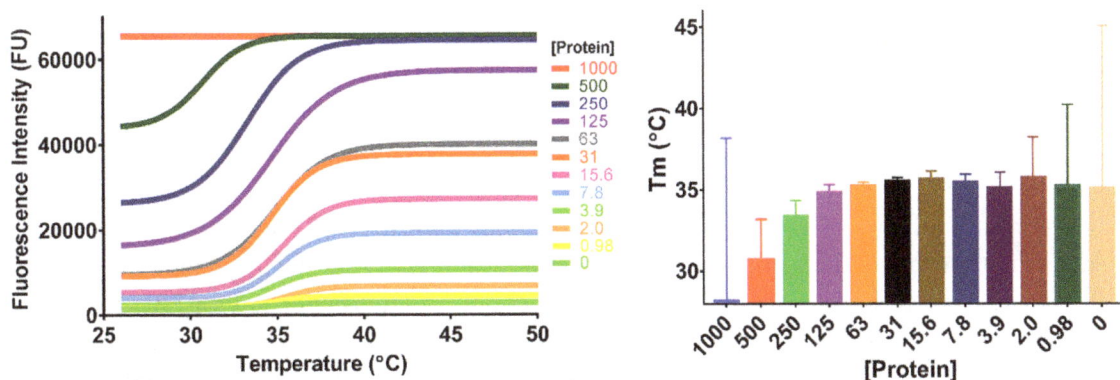

Figure 7. The importance of protein concentration in TSA. As protein concentration moves above or below the optimal range for the assay the curves fail to accurately represent the system and will increase the error of melting temperature calculation.

As in many fragment-screening assays, the quality of the library is paramount. In the assay development stage, a pilot assay should be run in which the concentration of solubilizing agent is varied over a range to define any effects that the agent might have on the stability of the protein. If time and availability of fragments allow, then a screen of fragment alone should be performed to check for fluorescence in the absence of ligand; this additional screen could yield data that is useful for removing problem compounds within the library. With an appropriate fragment library, it is possible to apply fragment to the screening plates. This is typically accomplished by using a pin tool or similar device capable of accurately delivering small volumes. After the plate has been exposed to the fragment library, it should be sealed with a fluorescently inert plate seal to avoid sample evaporation during the course of the assay. The assay plate should then be centrifuged to remove any air pockets from the samples, as these might reduce the quality of the data.

It has been established that TSA can be completed in a standard qPCR instrument [33]. The minimal requirement is the ability to evenly heat the samples over a suitable range of temperatures and record fluorescence. Deconvolution of resulting data output is variable based on instrumentation. This step can be time consuming and automation in data processing is helpful if large-scale projects are planned. Results should be recorded as fluorescent units recorded at each temperature in each well. This information can then be moved into data analysis software (e.g., *Graphpad Prism*, Graphpad Software, Inc.). Plotting fluorescence units against temperature should result in a sigmoidal curve reflecting the folded and unfolded states of the protein over a range of temperatures (**Figure 8a** and **b**). The signal commonly drops after it has reached a plateau. This drop is the result of aggregation in the protein-dye complex after denaturation [33]. Failure to remove data points resulting from this drop in signal can detrimentally affect subsequent curve fitting (**Figure 8a** and **b**). The Boltzmann equation can be adapted to calculate the exact T_m for each protein. Alternatively, it is possible to plot the derivative of the signal against temperature, recording the maximum of this derivative as the melting temperature (**Figure 8c**). The appropriate method for calculating the T_m can vary by target. Different methods should be tested to determine which calculation most accurately reflects the T_m of the experimental protein [32]. The thermal stability of a protein is increased to varying degrees when ligand is bound. The extent of this shift can vary greatly. In the case of fragment binding, thermal stabilization can be as little as 0.5 °C, making it crucial to establish the baseline stability of the protein within the experimental environment. It is then possible to establish the threshold of ΔT_m for a positive result in fragment stabilization of the ligand. As a rule of thumb, the standard deviation should not be greater than 10% of the ΔT_m [34].

There are many benefits to using TSA for the initial biophysical screening of a fragment library. First, the assay does not rely on the biochemical activity of the target and can be performed with limited knowledge of the target's function, which is beneficial for FBLD because fragment binding often does not yield a measurable biochemical result. Additionally, TSA requires only a small amount of minimally stable protein whose thermal stability can be tracked in the presence and absence of the ligand [30]. Thermal shift assays can be completed by using widely available RT-PCR instruments [33] and is relatively simple to perform with

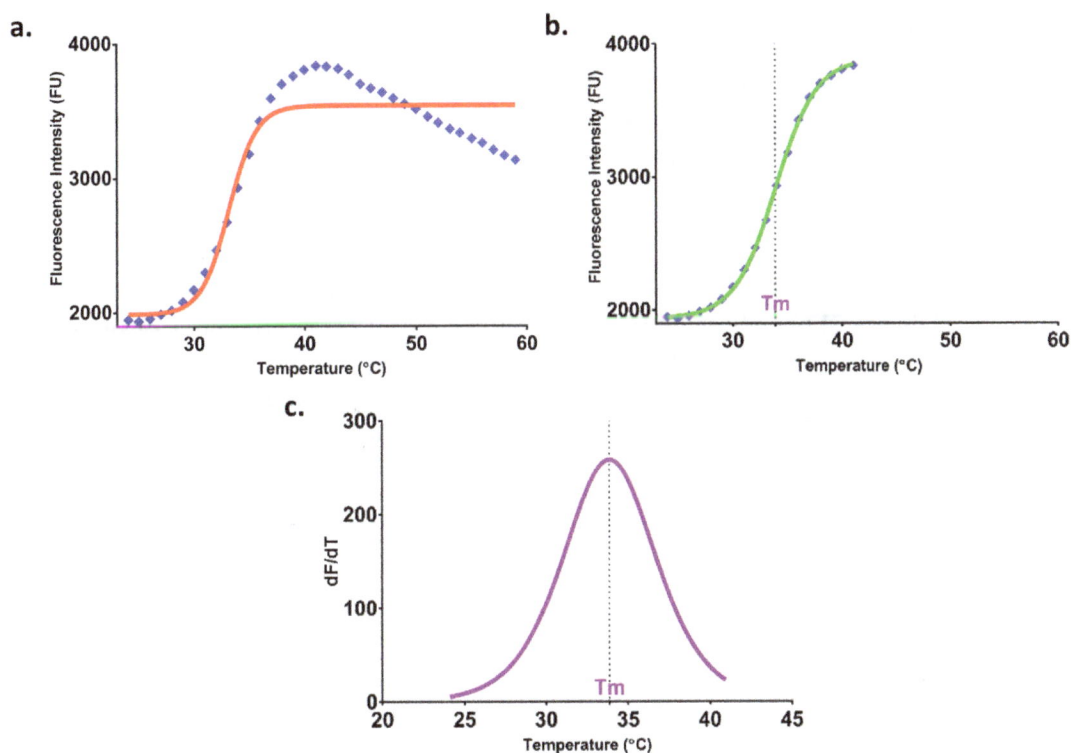

Figure 8. Curve fitting. (a) In this figure fluorescence intensity is plotted against temperature in blue. Above 41°C the dye begins to denature causing a decrease in signal. Fitting the full curve with the Boltzman equation (shown in red) would give an inaccurate estimation of T_m. (b) In this figure fluorescence intensity is plotted against temperature in blue. The data here is trimmed as signal begins to decrease improving the curve fitting (shown in green). (c) In this figure the change in fluorescence intensity over the change in temperature is plotted against temperature in purple.

limited training, reducing the up-front cost of implementing. This medium- to high-through-put assay typically enables the testing of up to 384 compounds in only 30–40 min.

Thermal shift assay is not a silver bullet *per se* and has some limitations and drawbacks. Traditional methods of assaying thermal shift will not work if a protein does not contain a hydrophobic core, as there will be nothing for the dye to differentially interact with when the target unfolds. Similarly, this assay will not produce valuable data if the surface of the protein is hydrophobic because the dye will fluoresce before the protein unfolds. Changing the dye used in the assay can mitigate these issues. The fluorescent readout of this assay also creates limitations. Some fragments commonly found in screening libraries fluoresce and interfere with the signal from SYPRO Orange. This phenomenon is readily evident upon inspection of the resulting data but requires a deconvolution step to avoid false-positive or false-negative results. Additionally, TSA does not provide accurate affinity data. However, a concentration versus ΔT_m curve can be fit to generate an EC_{50} value that can estimate the range in which subsequent biochemical or biophysical assays can be more effective [34, 35]. With these limitations in mind, TSA can be a powerful tool for detecting fragment binding.

3.5. Fragment validation

For the purposes of validation, a "good" fragment hit should be spatially described within a known target site via crystal structure, two-dimensional NMR studies, or at least, a ligand epitope map. The structural information enables the chemical expansion or linking of fragments during hit generation.

Hit rates in fragment-based screening are typically high, frequently at least an order of magnitude higher than those of ligand-based screening. Hits in the primary screen can be narrowed by using an orthogonal technique of comparable throughput for validation. Considering the numerous techniques available at the primary screening stage, the path to validation can be variable. Using an orthogonal approach to primary screening assumes that fragments that are hit by both techniques will translate successfully in secondary screening.

Using multiple techniques for fragment primary screening may yield a diminishing return. For example, after solving 71 crystal structures from soaking 361 fragments and statistically comparing the results of other fragment screening techniques [36], one group found that nearly half of the 71 "good" fragment hits were missed by other techniques. When used in combination, hit validation was statistically worse, but this fact was heightened by the inclusion of hits that were originally missed by crystallography. Therefore, orthogonal primary screening with at least two techniques still achieves the goal of fragment hit validation. However, if the primary fragment screening techniques do not provide meaningful structure characterization, then NMR or crystallography is required in a secondary screening capacity.

4. Fragment secondary screening

4.1. X-ray crystallography

Several companies, including Astex Pharmaceuticals, SGX Pharmaceuticals, Plexxikon, and Abbott, have effectively used structural biology in their fragment-based lead discovery efforts. This valuable tool avoids the pitfalls of false-positive results and nonspecific binding that may result from other fragment-screening methods. Any fragment hit discovered via crystallography is inherently validated for the given target. Crystallography gives a clear picture of the fragment binding posture within the active site. This information can greatly facilitate the design of libraries based on the initial hit.

Using crystallography as a method of fragment-based lead discovery has some limitations. It has long been associated with slow throughput. Additionally, some targets, such as membrane-associated proteins, do not readily lend themselves to crystallization. Crystallography often requires extensive and time-consuming efforts to arrive at crystallization conditions suitable for fragment soaking experiments. Even if these conditions have been determined, ready access to a suitable beam line and expertise in crystallography and data reduction can be hurdles in the rest of the lead discovery process. Protein in crystallization conditions is in a crystal lattice, which does not completely reflect a physiological environment. This artificial environment can lead to artifacts in the data and an inaccurate picture of fragment binding.

Although a crystal structure is rich in information, it does not reflect the potency or the biochemical activity of the bound fragment. With a wealth of structural information, it will not be possible to rank hits based on these criteria; orthogonal assays are critical for these purposes, and crystallography alone will not suffice.

The process of generating a fragment structure typically follows a set path. First, protein must be purified. Then, crystallization conditions for the purified protein are determined. Crystals can then either be grown in the presence of a fragment or soaked into a preexisting crystal. The resulting crystals are flash frozen and used for data collection either in house or at a larger beam line. The data is analyzed to generate a three-dimensional model of the fragment binding site within the target protein. This model can be used in iterative design efforts to grow the fragment into the binding site or link it to other fragments in neighboring sites.

Perhaps one of the most critical hurdles to successfully implementing structural biology into the FBLD process is having a suitable supply of the target protein. In most cases, protein used for X-ray crystallography must be pure and in high yields. A typical screen for crystallization conditions is completed by using as much as 20 mg/ml of protein. If initial crystal screening efforts using native protein are not effective, then it may be necessary to modify the target via removal of mobile loop regions or trimming the terminal ends. Creating multiple variants is commonly a valuable step in generating robust high-resolution structural data.

Once protein is available with sufficient yield and purity, screening for crystallization conditions begins. This is typically performed as a high-throughput screen with as many as 1000 set conditions in a single experiment. Many commercially available sparse matrix and additive crystallization screens use conditions that have historically yielded crystals. When these experiments yield a hit, the conditions can then be optimized to yield larger, highly reproducible crystals. Suitable crystals for fragment soaking should have fairly high resolution (<2 Å). Starting with a higher resolution structure improves resulting maps and increases the chances of producing an accurate model of fragment binding. If multiple crystallization conditions are available, it is best to choose the one that more closely represents physiological conditions, even at a slight cost to resolution. This trade-off will result in fragments with best chance of advancement to be prioritized.

Fragments suitable for X-ray crystallography benefit from good solubility, as insoluble fragments have a low probability of yielding a structure with suitable occupancy of the ligand. Compounds are soaked at high concentrations to improve the chances of high occupancy within the structure. Given this fact, a fragment should have a solubility of at least 1 mM [37]. SGX pharmaceuticals benefited from generating a brominated fragment library, which enabled detection of anomalous scatter as an indication of successful soaking, streamlining the data collection process. To further increase throughput, fragments were soaked in mixtures composed of fragments with diverse shapes. Resulting structures could then be deconvoluted based on the shape of the ligand in the active site [36]. Fragment mixtures do run the risk of decreasing the effective concentration of individual fragments in the mixture because high fragment concentration contributes to high-occupancy crystal structures, which can be detrimental to an experiment. In addition, these mixtures increase the chances of damaging the crystal in the soaking process, and fragments within the mix can interact with one another, skewing the results of the experiment. In one report, fragment mixtures resulted in 11 structures, whereas 20 structures resulted from individual soaking experiments [37]. These data suggest that if time and resources permit, soaking individual fragments is preferable to using mixtures.

If all other factors fall into place, a data set is collected. Improper treatment of this data set can result in an inaccurate and misleading model of fragment binding. Methods of data reduction and refinement are highly variable, and model building is a continuously evolving process. Certain steps in model building are especially pertinent when dealing with fragments. When searching for ligand density in a map, it is tempting to perform a quick refinement, and presume the location of a ligand. This approach is especially hazardous when modeling small fragments. If the map is not of high enough quality when the search for ligands begins, it is possible that water, a poorly resolved side chain, or even highly conserved buffers could masquerade as bound fragments [38]. It is best to perform several rounds of refinement before the ligand hunt begins. Model in any waters and then refine a few more times [37]. If the fragment is bound, a convincing map should take shape, and the creation of an accurate model of the target protein bound to fragments should be possible.

As technology progresses, many of the limitations of structural biology are being addressed. Most notably, throughput is being increased by incorporating automation. As this occurs, obtaining structural data is no longer the rate-limiting step in lead development. In several cases, automation of this process has improved to the extent that structural studies are successfully being used as a primary screen. Although this approach might not yet be a feasible option in laboratories with limited resources and limited access to beam lines, it holds promise for an improved fragment screening process in the future.

4.2. Isothermal titration calorimetry

Calorimetry measures the thermodynamics of a molecular interaction via observations of heat change in a reaction occurring in an adiabatic (thermodynamically closed) system [39]. In the context of drug discovery, the molecular interaction most commonly measured is the heat of binding of a small molecule to a protein target, although reaction kinetics can be measured under specific circumstances [40]. Measuring the heat associated with a molecular interaction allows direct measurement of the extent of breakage and formation of noncovalent interactions upon complex formation [39]. Using other methods, such as coupled reactions (e.g., product release) and fluorescent binding techniques, the change in enthalpy can only be inferred via the Van't Hoff relationship [41].

Classically, calorimetry has been applied to measurement of a binding interaction in two different ways: isothermal titration calorimetry, which measures heat release upon binding; and differential scanning calorimetry (DSC), which measures thermal stabilization of a protein due to binding of a small molecule. These methods offer a very detailed look at the thermodynamics of binding and have been used successfully in optimization after initial fragment hits have been identified. For the purposes of this chapter, discussion will be limited to ITC, as it is more directly applicable to FBDD. As a direct measurement of the heat of binding, ITC allows the researcher to remove the effects of fluorescent tags, antibody relationships, or coupling chemistry from the investigation of a binding relationship. Because ITC is a solution-based method, surface physical effects that interfere with binding (often seen with SPR) are not an issue.

Directly determining the thermodynamic components of overall binding allows a researcher to optimize a lead compound for a chosen target through specific binding interactions while minimizing off-target effects that often derail drug discovery programs. When combined with X-ray-based binding information or applied to analysis of structure-activity relationships, ITC can be a powerful tool in drug discovery. Overall binding of a small molecule to a target (as expressed by K_D) can be broken down into enthalpic (specific interactions such as H-bonding and π-stacking) and entropic (nonspecific events such as bound water release and increases in conformational flexibility) components.

The normal range of dissociation constants that can be measured by ITC is from 10 nM to 100 μM [41]. This range can be extended below 1 nM or above 1 mM by using displacement methods [42, 43], although a suitable displacement ligand (independently characterized) must be identified beforehand. Displacement ITC has not yet gained wide acceptance in drug discovery as of this writing, with most researchers reporting results of direct binding studies. Most fragments have binding affinities in the millimolar range, limiting the applicability of ITC as a screening method. In addition, large amounts of protein are typically required (usually 0.1–0.3 mg of protein per experiment, this moderate amount adds up for multiple samples and repeats). Each titration requires a moderate amount of time (45 min–1 h), but for a large number of samples, experiment time becomes a hurdle to using ITC as a screening method.

For these reasons, ITC is usually brought in to the drug discovery process after screening, as part of hit validation and lead optimization [44]. Fewer compounds are involved, allowing more focus on the large amount of information provided by ITC [44–46]. After a compound of interest is identified, a small set of structurally similar compounds can be purchased or synthesized to gain insight into the nature of binding to a target [47, 48]. At this stage, ITC offers the most benefit, as small molecules can be identified that maximize enthalpic interactions and minimize entropic interactions with the target.

Recent research into high-throughput calorimetry offer solutions to researchers wanting to incorporate calorimetry into an earlier stage in their screening cascade. Research into technologies in pursuit of the so-called "lab on a chip" has led to the development of both microfluidic [49] and droplet-based systems [50–52]. The droplet-based system has been applied to both binding and kinetics.

4.3. Fluorescence polarization

Biochemical screening is not a typical choice for the primary screening of fragments but can be used to verify an inhibition of function, and inhibition by a known mechanism which may help discriminate fragments binding to alternative target sites.

Fluorescence polarization-based assays are an option in FBDD when preliminary information about a target, such as small molecules that bind, is known. FP assays are competition assays in that they indirectly measure the effect of a compound on binding of an enzyme to a fluorescent probe. A fluorescent probe ideally starts out as a small molecule that binds tightly to an enzyme with known stoichiometry. This small molecule is chemically modified by the addition of a fluorescent label via an aliphatic or polyol linker to generate a fluorescent probe. Signal readout, represented in millipolarization units (mP), is calculated by measuring the amount of plane-polarized light passing through two filters (perpendicular and parallel to the plane of incident light) that remains after interaction with a solution containing probe and calculating the ratio of parallel to perpendicular light [53, 54]. In an FP assay, a plate reader measures the difference in relative tumbling between a free probe (high amount of tumbling, leading to more scattered emission, and thus low FP signal) and probe bound to a protein (low amount of tumbling, with more ordered emission relative to incident light, leading to high FP signal).

Depending on assay design, FP can be applied to either binding or activity assays, with ready-to-use kits available from BellBrook Labs [55] or Cayman Chemical [56]. Activity assays using FP rely on endpoint detection of binding to a probe, thus, are modified binding assays. For applications for which no kit is available, a small amount of synthesis can combine a small molecule of interest with a wide variety of synthetic fluorophores available from major vendors. When designing a probe for FP, resources such as the Molecular Probes Handbook [57] can be valuable.

FP is less commonly used in fragment screening than perhaps it should be. The range of binding affinities normally found in fragment libraries is in the high-μM to low-millimolar range, previously considered to be out of the range of FP when tight binding probes are used [58]. Although still somewhat limited in application by the need for a well-characterized probe, FP offers an inexpensive way to screen large numbers of compounds and has been used for many years in conventional drug discovery programs. With the advent of fragment-based techniques, FP is finding use both as a site directed primary [59, 60] and secondary [61–64] screening method, and has been used to validate new methods [65].

5. Fragment hit progression

For fragments, it is important to see activity in more than one assay, but equivalent potency in assays is not so important, and is not the best way to determine which molecules to promote. Various combinations of advanced metrics (i.e., efficiencies) with empirically driven evaluations (e.g., PAINS, metabolic stability) can help scientists make informed decisions on hit progression. An outside example of the successful application of metrics is sabermetrics. Today widely used in baseball, but also heavily scrutinized and evolving, sabermetrics uses advanced statistics to define in-game performance and improve decision-making by managers. Just like a game manager, scientists have to be aware of the limitations and effects of following a metric's indication, being consistent about hit progression occasionally in the light of conflicting results. Some experts [66] suggest using ligand efficiencies that can be easily determined without a calculator to facilitate discussions. Several metric-focused reviews are available to consult; one in particular covers a large number of reported hit-lead programs [67] for a wider perspective.

5.1. Empirically based fragment evaluations

Fragment screening methods virtually ensure that most screens will produce multiple hits for any target. Thus, the challenge to the researcher is not identifying compounds that interfere with a specific enzyme but determining which of many is the best to carry forward. Several metrics have emerged to guide the selection of fragment lead molecules through the drug discovery process: these metrics combine physical properties (e.g., molecular weight, cLogP, polar surface area, number of H-bond donors and acceptors) with potency data. The earliest of these was simply termed ligand efficiency (LE) and involved dividing the free energy (ΔG) of binding by the total number of nonhydrogen atoms in the molecule [68]. With the introduction of LE, researchers now havea relatively simple way to keep focused on the specificity of binding to the target, potentially avoiding downstream problems due to nonspecific binding [69].

Another metric in wide use in FBDD is lipophilic ligand efficiency (LLE) [70], which takes into account the total lipophilicity and potency of a molecule (IC_{50}, K_D, K_i). A useful modification of LLE (LLE_{Astex}) also controls for molecule size [71]. These statistical means of grading performance can support the early and late stages of the FBDD workflow and can be extended into progression analyses used during lead development (**Figure 9**). Which metric to use is up to the individual researcher and is based on the specific goals of the research program. Further reading to find an appropriate metric to use is recommended.

5.2. Hit generation

Fragments that progress to the hit-generation stage typically do so with structural insight that either describes the fragment bound to its protein target or the binding epitope mapped

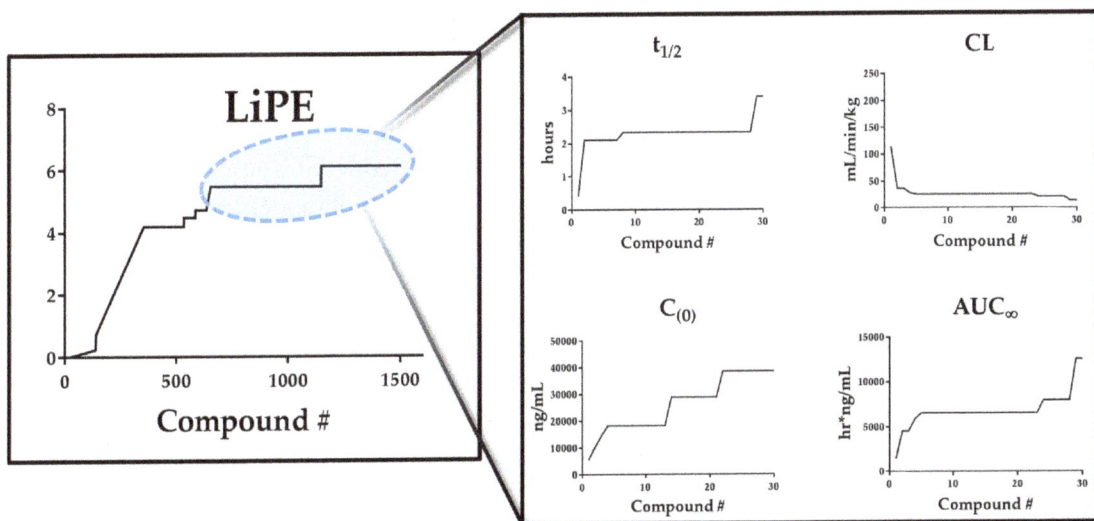

Figure 9. A typical progression analysis found in lead development can also include ligand efficiency metrics in a seamless fashion.

onto the fragment. A typical downstream workflow for hit generation includes a path that is structure blind, but this is essentially a diversion from traditional target-based discovery and may lead to an SAR bottleneck. The hit-generation stage refers to acquisition and screening of larger nonfragment ligands, which are obtained by catalog or synthetically prepared. This workflow includes either a chemical elaboration of individual fragments or the linking of at least two fragments, which then requires some optimization of the linker between them.

The hit generation phase is a practical place for virtual screening to be used to assist in fragment development. Method comparisons [72, 73] suggest that the currently available force fields and docking procedures based on lead-like molecules will provide adequate results for fragments (i.e., better than randomized screening). However, the careful consideration of a scoring function to reliably discern weak interactions cannot be overemphasized. Scientists have recognized this distinction within FBDD and have sought to improve the scoring functions for fragments [74]. One notable viewpoint is that fragment elaboration or linking may be facilitated when binding poses are expressed as Gibbs energy [75].

6. Conclusions

Considering that FBDD has been attributed to at least two FDA drug approvals, and that the platform is relatively easy to integrate into existing technologies, many companies and academic groups have started their own fragment-based discovery programs. The biophysical techniques each group uses will be dictated by the target, available facilities, and individual preferences of the investigators. Generally speaking, as long as the protein target has been successfully used with a technique in lead-like screening and structural information is available, there are virtually no other major obstacles to generating new chemical matter for a given target-based screening program. What remains are practical challenges, two of which bear repeating for those who are in the beginning stages of FBDD.

First, the key practical difference between lead-like screening and fragment screening is the use of high concentrations of the fragments. The increased concentration impacts the compound library that is used and the clarity at which hits are delineated. Some suggestions have been made as to the optimal concentrations to use for a given technique. These are only suggestions and will likely change based on the system and techniques employed. With some practice, these procedures can be suitably optimized and need less attention going forward.

Second, is the challenge of directing fragment build out and/or fragment linking chemistry which can be resource intensive. As such, medicinal chemists are aided by the use of a preferred ligand efficiency metric early in the FBDD process to assist the ranking of fragment hits. Certainly other empirical and nonempirical factors will influence the progression of fragments, but metrics will help organize the structure-activity relationship which is a key driver of the expansion or linking of fragments during hit generation.

Acknowledgments

The authors would like to acknowledge the funding support from the National Institutes of Health grant R01AI110578, and the American Lebanese Syrian Associated Charities (ALSAC), St Jude Children's Research Hospital. We thank Cherise Guess, PhD, ELS, of the SJCRH Department of Scientific Editing for her assistance with editing.

Author details

John J. Bowling[1], William R. Shadrick[1], Elizabeth C. Griffith[1] and Richard E. Lee[1, 2]*

*Address all correspondence to: Richard.Lee@stjude.org

1 Department of Chemical Biology and Therapeutics, St. Jude Children's Research Hospital, Memphis, TN, United States

2 Department of Pharmaceutical Sciences, University of Tennessee Health Science Center, Memphis, TN, United States

References

[1] Macarron R, Banks MN, Bojanic D, Burns DJ, Cirovic DA, Garyantes T, Green DVS, Hertzberg RP, Janzen WP, Paslay JW, Schopfer U, Sittampalam GS. Impact of high-throughput screening in biomedical research. Nat Rev Drug Discov. 2011; 10(3): 188–95. DOI: 10.1038/nrd3368

[2] Reymond J-L. The chemical space project. Acc Chem Res. 2015; 48(3): 722–30. DOI: 10.1021/ar500432k

[3] Hert J, Irwin JJ, Laggner C, Keiser MJ, Shoichet BK. Quantifying biogenic bias in screening libraries. Nat Chem Biol. 2009; 5(7): 479–83. DOI: 10.1038/nchembio.180

[4] Hann MM, Leach AR, Harper G. Molecular complexity and its impact on the probability of finding leads for drug discovery. J Chem Inf Comp Sci. 2001; 41(3): 856–64. DOI: 10.1021/ci000403i

[5] Jencks WP. On the attribution and additivity of binding energies. Proc Natl Acad Sci USA. 1981; 78(7): 4046–50. DOI: N/A

[6] Shuker SB, Hajduk PJ, Meadows RP, Fesik SW. Discovering high-affinity ligands for proteins: SAR by NMR. Science. 1996; 274(5292): 1531–4. DOI: 10.1126/science.274.5292.1531

[7] Bollag G, Tsai J, Zhang J, Zhang C, Ibrahim P, Nolop K, Hirth P. Vemurafenib: the first drug approved for BRAF-mutant cancer. Nat Rev Drug Discov. 2012; 11(11): 873–86. DOI: 10.1038/nrd3847

[8]   Deeks ED. Venetoclax: first global approval. Drugs. 2016; 76(9): 979–87. DOI: 10.1007/
      s40265-016-0596-x

[9]   Erlanson DA, Fesik SW, Hubbard RE, Jahnke W, Jhoti H. Twenty years on: the impact of
      fragments on drug discovery. Nat Rev Drug Discov. 2016; 15(9): 605–19. DOI: 10.1038/
      nrd.2016.109

[10] Congreve M, Carr R, Murray C, Jhoti H. A 'Rule of Three' for fragment-based lead dis-
      covery? Drug Discov Today. 2003; 8(19): 876–7. DOI: 10.1016/S1359-6446(03)02831-9

[11] Jhoti H, Williams G, Rees DC, Murray CW. The 'rule of three' for fragment-based drug
      discovery: where are we now? Nat Rev Drug Discov. 2013; 12(8): 644. DOI: 10.1038/
      nrd3926-c1

[12] Keseru GM, Erlanson DA, Ferenczy GG, Hann MM, Murray CW, Pickett SD. Design
      principles for fragment libraries: maximizing the value of learnings from pharma frag-
      ment-based drug discovery (FBDD) programs for use in academia. J Med Chem. 2016;
      59(18): 8189–206. DOI: 10.1021/acs.jmedchem.6b00197

[13] Swain C. Fragment Collections [Internet]. 2016. Available from: http://www.cam-
      bridgemedchemconsulting.com/resources/hit_identification/fragment_collections.html
      [Accessed: 2016-09-09]

[14] Lau WF, Withka JM, Hepworth D, Magee TV, Du YJ, Bakken GA, Miller MD, Hendsch ZS,
      Thanabal V, Kolodziej SA, Xing L, Hu Q, Narasimhan LS, Love R, Charlton ME, Hughes
      S, van Hoorn WP, Mills JE. Design of a multi-purpose fragment screening library using
      molecular complexity and orthogonal diversity metrics. J Comput Aid Mol Des. 2011;
      25(7): 621–36. DOI: 10.1007/s10822-011-9434-0

[15] Kutchukian PS, So S-S, Fischer C, Waller CL. Fragment library design: using cheminfor-
      matics and expert chemists to fill gaps in existing fragment libraries. In: Klon EA, editor.
      Fragment-Based Methods in Drug Discovery. New York, NY: Springer New York; 2015.
      pp. 43–53. DOI: 10.1007/978-1-4939-2486-8_5

[16] Davis BJ, Erlanson DA. Learning from our mistakes: the 'unknown knowns' in fragment
      screening. Bioorg Med Chem Lett. 2013; 23(10): 2844–52. DOI: 10.1016/j.bmcl.2013.03.028

[17] Lagorce D, Sperandio O, Baell JB, Miteva MA, Villoutreix BO. FAF-Drugs3: a web server
      for compound property calculation and chemical library design. Nucleic Acid Res. 2015;
      43(W1): W200–W7. DOI: 10.1093/nar/gkv353

[18] Mayer M, Meyer B. Group epitope mapping by saturation transfer difference NMR to
      identify segments of a ligand in direct contact with a protein receptor. J Am Chem Soc.
      2001; 123(25): 6108–17. DOI: 10.1021/ja0100120

[19] Sledz P, Silvestre HL, Hung AW, Ciulli A, Blundell TL, Abell C. Optimization of the
      interligand Overhauser effect for fragment linking: application to inhibitor discovery
      against mycobacterium tuberculosis pantothenate synthetase. J Am Chem Soc. 2010;
      132(13): 4544–5. DOI: 10.1021/ja100595u

[20] Vanwetswinkel S, Heetebrij RJ, van Duynhoven J, Hollander JG, Filippov DV, Hajduk PJ, Siegal G. TINS, Target immobilized NMR screening: an efficient and sensitive method for ligand discovery. Chem Biol. 2005; 12(2): 207–16. DOI: 10.1016/j.chembiol.2004.12.004

[21] Gardner KH, Kay LE. Production and incorporation of 15N, 13C, 2H (1H-δ1 methyl) iso-leucine into proteins for multidimensional NMR studies. J Am Chem Soc. 1997; 119(32): 7599–600. DOI: 10.1021/ja9706514

[22] Hajduk PJ, Augeri DJ, Mack J, Mendoza R, Yang J, Betz SF, Fesik SW. NMR-Based screen-ing of proteins containing 13C-labeled methyl groups. J Am Chem Soc. 2000; 122(33): 7898–904. DOI: 10.1021/ja000350l

[23] Dalvit C. Ligand- and substrate-based 19F NMR screening: principles and applica-tions to drug discovery. Prog Nucl Mag Res Sp. 2007; 51(4): 243–71. DOI: 10.1016/j.pnmrs.2007.07.002

[24] Rich RL, Myszka DG. Survey of the 2009 commercial optical biosensor literature. J Mol Recognit. 2011; 24(6): 892–914. DOI: 10.1002/jmr.1138

[25] Johnsson B, Löfås S, Lindquist G. Immobilization of proteins to a carboxymethyldex-tran-modified gold surface for biospecific interaction analysis in surface plasmon reso-nance sensors. Anal Biochem. 1991; 198(2): 268–77. DOI: 10.1016/0003-2697(91)90424-R

[26] Rich RL, Quinn JG, Morton T, Stepp JD, Myszka DG. Biosensor-based fragment screening using FastStep injections. Anal Biochem. 2010; 407(2): 270–7. DOI: 10.1016/j.ab.2010.08.024

[27] Karlsson R, Katsamba PS, Nordin H, Pol E, Myszka DG. Analyzing a kinetic titration series using affinity biosensors. Anal Biochem. 2006; 349(1): 136–47. DOI: 10.1016/j.ab.2005.09.034

[28] Quinn JG. Evaluation of Taylor dispersion injections: determining kinetic/affinity inter-action constants and diffusion coefficients in label-free biosensing. Anal Biochem. 2012; 421(2): 401–10. DOI: 10.1016/j.ab.2011.11.023

[29] Quinn JG. Modeling Taylor dispersion injections: determination of kinetic/affinity inter-action constants and diffusion coefficients in label-free biosensing. Anal Biochem. 2012; 421(2): 391–400. DOI: 10.1016/j.ab.2011.11.024

[30] Pantoliano MW, Petrella EC, Kwasnoski JD, Lobanov VS, Myslik J, Graf E, Carver T, Asel E, Springer BA, Lane P, Salemme FR. High-density miniaturized thermal shift assays as a general strategy for drug discovery. J Biomol Screen. 2001; 6(6): 429–40. DOI: 10.1089/108705701753364922

[31] Ciulli A. Biophysical screening for the discovery of small-molecule ligands. In: Williams M, Daviter T, editors. Methods in Molecular Biology. 2nd ed. New York: Springer; 2013. pp. 357–88. DOI: 10.1007/978-1-62703-398-5_13

[32] Schiebel J, Radeva N, Koster H, Metz A, Krotzky T, Kuhnert M, Diederich WE, Heine A, Neumann L, Atmanene C, Roecklin D, Vivat-Hannah V, Renaud JP, Meinecke R, Schlinck

N, Sitte A, Popp F, Zeeb M, Klebe G. One question, multiple answers: biochemical and biophysical screening methods retrieve deviating fragment hit lists. Chemmedchem. 2015; 10(9): 1511–21. DOI: 10.1002/cmdc.201500267

[33] Lo MC, Aulabaugh A, Jin G, Cowling R, Bard J, Malamas M, Ellestad G. Evaluation of fluorescence-based thermal shift assays for hit identification in drug discovery. Anal Biochem. 2004; 332(1): 153–9. DOI: 10.1016/j.ab.2004.04.031

[34] Vivoli M, Novak HR, Littlechild JA, Harmer NJ. Determination of protein-ligand interactions using differential scanning fluorimetry. J Vis Exp. 2014; 91: 51809. DOI: 10.3791/51809

[35] Groftehauge MK, Hajizadeh NR, Swann MJ, Pohl E. Protein-ligand interactions investigated by thermal shift assays (TSA) and dual polarization interferometry (DPI). Acta Crystallogr D. 2015; 71(Pt 1): 36–44. DOI: 10.1107/S1399004714016617

[36] Schiebel J, Radeva N, Krimmer SG, Wang X, Stieler M, Ehrmann FR, Fu K, Metz A, Huschmann FU, Weiss MS, Mueller U, Heine A, Klebe G. Six biophysical screening methods miss a large proportion of crystallographically discovered fragment hits: a case study. ACS Chem Biol. 2016; 11(6): 1693–701. DOI: 10.1021/acschembio.5b01034

[37] Schiebel J, Krimmer SG, Rower K, Knorlein A, Wang X, Park AY, Stieler M, Ehrmann FR, Fu K, Radeva N, Krug M, Huschmann FU, Glockner S, Weiss MS, Mueller U, Klebe G, Heine A. High-throughput crystallography: reliable and efficient identification of fragment hits. Structure. 2016; 24(8): 1398–409. DOI: 10.1016/j.str.2016.06.010

[38] Kleywegt GJ. Crystallographic refinement of ligand complexes. Acta Crystallogr D. 2007; 63(Pt 1): 94–100. DOI: 10.1107/S0907444906022657

[39] Ladbury JE, Klebe G, Freire E. Adding calorimetric data to decision making in lead discovery: a hot tip. Nat Rev Drug Discov. 2010; 9(1): 23–7. DOI: 10.1038/nrd3054

[40] Hansen LD, Transtrum MK, Quinn C, Demarse N. Enzyme-catalyzed and binding reaction kinetics determined by titration calorimetry. Biochim Biophys Acta. 2016; 1860(5): 957–66. DOI: 10.1016/j.bbagen.2015.12.018

[41] Ladbury JE. Calorimetry as a tool for understanding biomolecular interactions and an aid to drug design. Biochem Soc T. 2010; 38(4): 888–93. DOI: 10.1042/bst0380888

[42] Velazquez-Campoy A, Freire E. Isothermal titration calorimetry to determine association constants for high-affinity ligands. Nat Protoc. 2006; 1(1): 186–91. DOI: 10.1038/nprot.2006.28

[43] Ruhmann E, Betz M, Fricke M, Heine A, Schafer M, Klebe G. Thermodynamic signatures of fragment binding: validation of direct versus displacement ITC titrations. Biochim Biophys Acta. 2015; 1850(4): 647–56. DOI: 10.1016/j.bbagen.2014.12.007

[44] Mashalidis EH, Sledz P, Lang S, Abell C. A three-stage biophysical screening cascade for fragment-based drug discovery. Nat Protoc. 2013; 8(11): 2309–24. DOI: 10.1038/nprot.2013.130

[45] Ladbury JE. Isothermal titration calorimetry: application to structure-based drug design. Thermochim Acta. 2001; 380(2): 209–15. DOI: 10.1016/S0040-6031(01)00674-8

[46] Scott DE, Ehebauer MT, Pukala T, Marsh M, Blundell TL, Venkitaraman AR, Abell C, Hyvonen M. Using a fragment-based approach to target protein-protein interactions. Chembiochem. 2013; 14(3): 332–42. DOI: 10.1002/cbic.201200521

[47] Banerjee DR, Dutta D, Saha B, Bhattacharyya S, Senapati K, Das AK, Basak A. Design, synthesis and characterization of novel inhibitors against mycobacterial beta-ketoacyl CoA reductase FabG4. Org Biomol Chem. 2014; 12(1): 73–85. DOI: 10.1039/c3ob41676c

[48] Kišonaite M, Zubriene A, Čapkauskaite E, Smirnov A, Smirnoviene J, Kairys V, Michailoviene V, Manakova E, Gražulis S, Matulis D. Intrinsic thermodynamics and structure correlation of benzenesulfonamides with a pyrimidine moiety binding to carbonic anhydrases I, II, VII, XII, and XIII. Plos One. 2014; 9(12): e114106. DOI: 10.1371/journal.pone.0114106

[49] Wolf A, Hartmann T, Bertolini M, Schemberg J, Grodrian A, Lemke K, Förster T, Kessler E, Hänschke F, Mertens F, Paus R, Lerchner J. Toward high-throughput chip calorimetry by use of segmented-flow technology. Thermochim Acta. 2015; 603: 172–83. DOI: 10.1016/j.tca.2014.10.021

[50] Recht MI, Nienaber V, Torres FE. Fragment-based screening for enzyme inhibitors using calorimetry. Method Enzymol. 2016; 567: 47–69. DOI: 10.1016/bs.mie.2015.07.023

[51] Recht MI, Sridhar V, Badger J, Bounaud PY, Logan C, Chie-Leon B, Nienaber V, Torres FE. Identification and optimization of PDE10A inhibitors using fragment-based screening by nanocalorimetry and X-ray crystallography. J Biomol Screen. 2014; 19(4): 497–507. DOI: 10.1177/1087057113516493

[52] Torres FE, Kuhn P, De Bruyker D, Bell AG, Wolkin MV, Peeters E, Williamson JR, Anderson GB, Schmitz GP, Recht MI, Schweizer S, Scott LG, Ho JH, Elrod SA, Schultz PG, Lerner RA, Bruce RH. Enthalpy arrays. Proc Natl Acad Sci U S A. 2004; 101(26): 9517–22. DOI: 10.1073/pnas.0403573101

[53] Lea WA, Simeonov A. Fluorescence polarization assays in small molecule screening. Expert Opin Drug Discov. 2011; 6(1): 17–32. DOI: 10.1517/17460441.2011.537322

[54] Rossi AM, Taylor CW. Analysis of protein-ligand interactions by fluorescence polarization. Nat Protoc. 2011; 6(3): 365–87. DOI: 10.1038/nprot.2011.305

[55] BellBrook Labs. Transcreener® HTS Assays [Internet]. 2016. Available from: https://www.bellbrooklabs.com/products-services/transcreener-hts-assays/[Accessed: 2016-09-23]

[56] Cayman Chemical. Assay Kits [Internet]. 2016. Available from: https://www.cayman-chem.com/Products/kits [Accessed: 2016-09-23]

[57] Thermo Fisher Scientific. The Molecular Probes Handbook [Internet]. 2016. Available from: http://www.thermofisher.com/us/en/home/references/molecular-probes-the-handbook.html [Accessed: 2016-09-23]

[58] Xinyi H. Fluorescence polarization competition assay: the range of resolvable inhibitor potency is limited by the affinity of the fluorescent ligand. J Biomol Screen. 2003; 8(1): 34–8. DOI: 10.1177/1087057102239666

[59] Baughman BM, Jake Slavish P, DuBois RM, Boyd VA, White SW, Webb TR. Identification of influenza endonuclease inhibitors using a novel fluorescence polarization assay. ACS Chem Biol. 2012; 7(3): 526–34. DOI: 10.1021/cb200439z

[60] Carson MW, Zhang J, Chalmers MJ, Bocchinfuso WP, Holifield KD, Masquelin T, Stites RE, Stayrook KR, Griffin PR, Dodge JA. HDX reveals unique fragment ligands for the vitamin D receptor. Bioorg Med Chem Lett. 2014; 24(15): 3459–63. DOI: 10.1016/j.bmcl.2014.05.070

[61] Davies NGM, Browne H, Davis B, Drysdale MJ, Foloppe N, Geoffrey S, Gibbons B, Hart T, Hubbard R, Jensen MR, Mansell H, Massey A, Matassova N, Moore JD, Murray J, Pratt R, Ray S, Robertson A, Roughley SD, Schoepfer J, Scriven K, Simmonite H, Stokes S, Surgenor A, Webb P, Wood M, Wright L, Brough P. Targeting conserved water molecules: design of 4-aryl-5-cyanopyrrolo[2,3-d]pyrimidine Hsp90 inhibitors using fragment-based screening and structure-based optimization. Bioorg Med Chem. 2012; 20(22): 6770–89. DOI: 10.1016/j.bmc.2012.08.050

[62] Yin Z, Whittell LR, Wang Y, Jergic S, Liu M, Harry EJ, Dixon NE, Beck JL, Kelso MJ, Oakley AJ. Discovery of lead compounds targeting the bacterial sliding clamp using a fragment-based approach. J Med Chem. 2014; 57(6): 2799–806. DOI: 10.1021/jm500122r

[63] Yu W, Xiao H, Lin J, Li C. Discovery of novel STAT3 small molecule inhibitors via in silico site-directed fragment-based drug design. J Med Chem. 2013; 56(11): 4402–12. DOI: 10.1021/jm400080c

[64] Zhao L, Cao D, Chen T, Wang Y, Miao Z, Xu Y, Chen W, Wang X, Li Y, Du Z, Xiong B, Li J, Xu C, Zhang N, He J, Shen J. Fragment-based drug discovery of 2-thiazolidinones as inhibitors of the histone reader BRD4 bromodomain. J Med Chem. 2013; 56(10): 3833–51. DOI: 10.1021/jm301793a

[65] Meiby E, Simmonite H, le Strat L, Davis B, Matassova N, Moore JD, Mrosek M, Murray J, Hubbard RE, Ohlson S. Fragment screening by weak affinity chromatography: comparison with established techniques for screening against HSP90. Anal Chem. 2013; 85(14): 6756–66. DOI: 10.1021/ac400715t

[66] Zartler E. Practical Fragments [Internet]. Erlanson D, editor. Blogger: Google Inc. 2015. [2016/08/01]. Available from: http://practicalfragments.blogspot.com/2015/09/is-this-still-thing-and-why.html

[67] Ferenczy GG, Keseru GM. How are fragments optimized? A retrospective analysis of 145 fragment optimizations. J Med Chem. 2013; 56(6): 2478–86. DOI: 10.1021/jm301851v

[68] Hopkins AL, Groom CR, Alex A. Ligand efficiency: a useful metric for lead selection. Drug Discov Today. 2004; 9(10): 430–1. DOI: 10.1016/s1359-6446(04)03069-7

[69] Hughes JP, Rees S, Kalindjian SB, Philpott KL. Principles of early drug discovery. Brit J Pharmacol. 2011; 162(6): 1239–49. DOI: 10.1111/j.1476-5381.2010.01127.x

[70] Leeson PD, Springthorpe B. The influence of drug-like concepts on decision-making in medicinal chemistry. Nat Rev Drug Discov. 2007; 6(11): 881–90. DOI: 10.1038/nrd2445

[71] Mortenson PN, Murray CW. Assessing the lipophilicity of fragments and early hits. J Comput Aid Mol Des. 2011; 25(7): 663–7. DOI: 10.1007/s10822-011-9435-z

[72] Kawatkar S, Wang H, Czerminski R, Joseph-McCarthy D. Virtual fragment screening: an exploration of various docking and scoring protocols for fragments using Glide. J Comput Aid Mol Des. 2009; 23(8): 527–39. DOI: 10.1007/s10822-009-9281-4

[73] Sándor M, Kiss R, Keseru GM. Virtual fragment docking by glide: a validation study on 190 protein-fragment complexes. J Chem Inf Model. 2010; 50(6): 1165–72. DOI: 10.1021/ci1000407

[74] Wang J-C, Lin J-H. Scoring functions for prediction of protein-ligand interactions. Curr Pharm Design. 2013; 19(12): 2174–82. DOI: 10.2174/1381612811319120005

[75] Kozakov D, Hall DR, Jehle S, Luo L, Ochiana SO, Jones EV, Pollastri M, Allen KN, Whitty A, Vajda S. Ligand deconstruction: why some fragment binding positions are conserved and others are not. Proc Nat Acad Sci. 2015; 112(20): E2585–E94. DOI: 10.1073/pnas.1501567112

2

Chemical Similarity Networks for Drug Discovery

Yu-Chen Lo and Jorge Z. Torres

Additional information is available at the end of the chapter

Abstract

Chemical similarity networks are an emerging area of interest in medicinal chemistry, chemical biology, and systems chemoinformatics that are currently being applied to drug target prediction, drug repurposing, and drug discovery in the new paradigm of poly-pharmacology and systems biology. In this chapter, we discuss the network-based drug target identification and discovery framework called chemical similarity network analysis pull-down (CSNAP) and its applications. We highlight the utility of CSNAP in identifying novel antimitotic drugs and their targets through practical case studies.

Keywords: drug discovery, chemical similarity networks, target identification

1. Introduction

Chemical similarity is an important concept in drug discovery used to identify compounds with similar bioactivities based on structural similarity between two ligands [1, 2]. Once a lead compound has been discovered from a chemical screen, a drug designer can design a series of structural analogues with improved pharmaceutical properties. The fundamental principle behind similarity-based drug discovery is the "chemical similarity principle," which states that if two molecules share similar structures, then they will likely have similar bioactivities. While there are exceptions, correlation between chemical structure and compound activities has been well established in medicinal chemistry [3]. Consequently, determining whether two molecules are structurally similar is a prerequisite for similarity-based drug discovery. At a rudimentary level, the similarity between two ligands can be easily discerned through visual inspection by identifying common functional groups, structural motifs, or substructures. However, human intervention is often subjective and not suitable for large-scale analysis.

Thus, applying computational algorithms for unbiased chemical similarity comparison and database searching is essential for a successful drug discovery campaign.

Several computational chemical similarity search algorithms have been developed [1, 4, 5]. The most commonly used approaches use chemical substructure fingerprints. Non-hashed structural fingerprints such as MACCS keys or Obabel FP3 fingerprints detect predefined substructures or functional group patterns in a molecule by mapping common chemical motifs into binary arrays known as structural keys. To compare the chemical similarity between two molecules, each molecule is converted into a binary series of 0 and 1, indicating the absence and presence of a particular substructure. On the other hand, chemical hashed fingerprints such as Daylight fingerprints or Obabel FP2 fingerprints use path information derived from molecular graphs to compare chemical structures [4]. While path-based fingerprints usually confer higher specificity, structural fingerprints can nevertheless be useful for detecting hits with distinct chemical scaffolds. Once the chemical fingerprints have been determined in a chemical search and the molecules have been converted to appropriate data representations, the next step is to evaluate the chemical similarity using a distance metric. Common distance measures include Euclidean, Manhattan, and Mahalanobis metrics, which have been widely applied in chemoinformatics and bioinformatics applications [6]. However, in the case of binary chemical fingerprints, the simplest and most direct distance measure is the Tanimoto index. Tanimoto metrics calculate the fraction of shared bits between chemical fingerprints in the range of 0–1. Although there is no universal Tanimoto index cutoff (Tc) to determine whether two molecules are sufficiently similar, a Tc value of 0.7 is a reasonable starting point for most chemical searches. Alternatively, statistical scores such as a Z-score can also be calculated based on the overall Tc score distribution [7].

In addition to 2D fingerprints, 3D chemical similarity fingerprints have also been developed. 3D chemical similarity fingerprints utilize the 3D structural information of the ligands such as molecular shape, pharmacophore points, or molecular interaction fields (MIF) for structural similarity comparison. Although 3D chemical similarity comparison can often capture structural features essential for protein-ligand binding, 3D alignment algorithms often require extensive optimization procedures to maximize the overlapped volume and are computationally intensive. Alternatively, nonalignment methods based on chemical descriptors such as GETAWAY or 3D-MoRSE descriptors can also be used [8, 9]. The 3D chemical descriptor is capable of capturing 3D ligand properties from 2D information and may improve computational time. However, substantial postvalidation may be required to confirm 3D structural similarity.

2. Network-based target prediction and drug discovery

The application of chemical similarity searches for ligand bioactivity prediction has recently gained substantial interest [10]. Due to the high failure rate of many new chemical entities (NCE) in the late stage of clinical trials, understanding on- and off-target binding of a drug to predict mechanisms of action and adverse reactions has become crucial for drug discovery programs [11]. If the chemical structure of a compound is known, then it is possible to predict compound bioactivities based on the chemical similarity methods described previously. Drug targets can be inferred from bioactivity databases with annotated targets sharing the highest similarity to the target molecules. Many public bioactivity databases are freely available and can be applied to this application including ChEMBL, PubChem, DrugBank, and Binding Database to name a few [12–14].

The simplest approach for drug target inference is by a simple chemical similarity search where the target of a query compound is inferred from the annotated ligand sharing the highest chemical similarity (**Figure 1**). However, there are several limitations to this approach. First, target information for the reference molecules may be incomplete; thus, target inference from a single molecular entity can miss potential targets from molecules sharing lower chemical similarity. Likewise, pair-wise target predictions may not provide consistent predictions for a group of structurally similar ligands. Second, chemical similarity values are not effective at ranking on and off targets and do not consider the structure-activity relationship (SAR) of congeneric series. Most importantly, simple ligand-based searches cannot be applied to analyzing large numbers of ligands such as the unannotated hits from a chemical screen. To circumvent this shortcoming, we recently proposed a new network target inference approach based on chemical similarity networks called chemical similarity network analysis pull-down (CSNAP) [15].

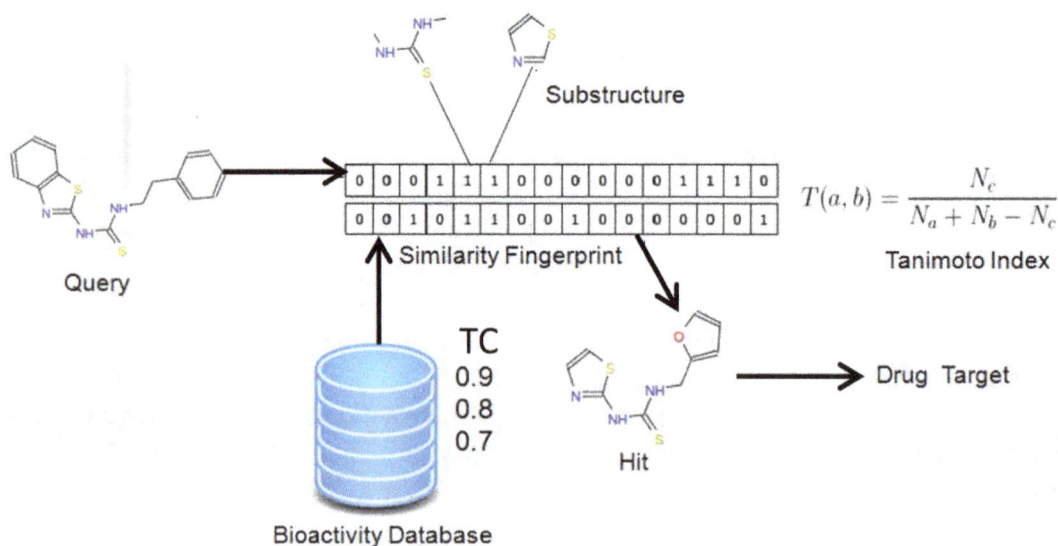

$$T(a, b) = \frac{N_c}{N_a + N_b - N_c}$$

Tanimoto Index

Figure 1. Chemical similarity search using 2D chemical fingerprints.

CSNAP uses a network-based algorithm to predict drug targets and does not rely on absolute chemical similarity values. It utilizes a scoring function (S-score) to find the consensus targets of a ligand in its nearest neighbors in a chemical similarity network, which is similar to that used to predict protein functions in a protein-protein interaction (PPI) network [16]. CSNAP is compatible with publicly available bioactivity databases, and we routinely use the ChEMBL database, which is one of the largest bioactivity databases that contains more than 1 million compounds with known target annotations. The original CSNAP algorithm applies 2D Obabel chemical similarity fingerprints (FP2, FP3, FP4, and MACCS) for target predictions. More recently, we developed CSNAP3D that combines 2D and 3D chemical search algorithms to improve the chemical search space [17]. CSNAP3D uses a fast 2D chemical similarity search using either FP2 or FP3 fingerprints to identify sets of hit molecules from large compound databases, and hit molecules are rescored using a combination of 3D similarity descriptors based on a combination of shape and pharmacophore. From our benchmark studies, we found that the CSNAP computational framework was highly accurate and was capable of analyzing large compound sets with diverse chemical structures. Consistently, the CSNAP application has been recently extended for large-scale metabolite analysis [18]. We have made the CSNAP algorithm freely available as the CSNAP web and it can be accessed at http://services.mbi.ucla.edu/CSNAP/.

3. CSNAP implementation

3.1. Chemical similarity network algorithms

Mathematically, a chemical similarity network can be considered as a graph G (V, E) where the vertex V represents compounds and the edge E represents chemical similarity and connects two compounds if they share a chemical similarity above an arbitrary threshold [19]. The CSNAP algorithm is performed in three steps: (1) chemical similarity database search, (2) chemical similarity network construction, and (3) drug target scoring and inference.

3.1.1. Chemical similarity search

Chemical similarity searching is the first step in the CSNAP algorithm (**Figure 2A**). The chemical similarity comparisons are performed using various 2D Obabel fingerprints including FP2, FP3, MACCS, and others. Query compounds prepared in SMILES or SDF formats are used as inputs to the CSNAP program. The compounds are searched sequentially against the ChEMBL database. To identify the ChEMBL compounds most similar to the query, the relative chemical similarity score is quantified by a Z-value relative to the distribution of the top 100 chemical similarity values. The ChEMBL compounds with a Z-score >2.5 are selected and serve as the annotated compounds for target inference in the next step.

3.1.2. Chemical similarity network construction

To generate chemical similarity networks, pair-wise chemical similarity values are evaluated between every pair of compounds. A network edge is established between two ligands whenever their similarity value is above a predefined threshold (>0.7) (**Figure 2B**). When large compound data sets are analyzed by the CSNAP algorithm, structurally diverse compounds are partitioned into subnetworks of distinct chemical scaffolds, known as "chemotypes." The chemical similarity networks can be used to estimate the chemical diversity of input structures at this stage.

3.1.3. Drug target scoring and inference

CSNAP infers drug targets using consensus statistics. Specifically, drug targets in the first neighbor of the query are identified and ranked based on their target annotation frequency (**Figure 2C**). A consensus score called an S-score is used to rank the probability that the predicted target will interact with the query ligand (**Figure 2D**). There are several advantages of using this network-based scoring function. First, the S-score eliminates the possibility of missing target information from the nearest neighbor and considers all possible targets within the same congeneric series. Second, since the drug target is inferred from the target consensus and is in agreement with the observed structure-activity relationship, the robustness of the prediction increases substantially. From our benchmark studies, we showed that this network-based target inference approach improves the prediction success rate over traditional approaches that use simple chemical searches [15].

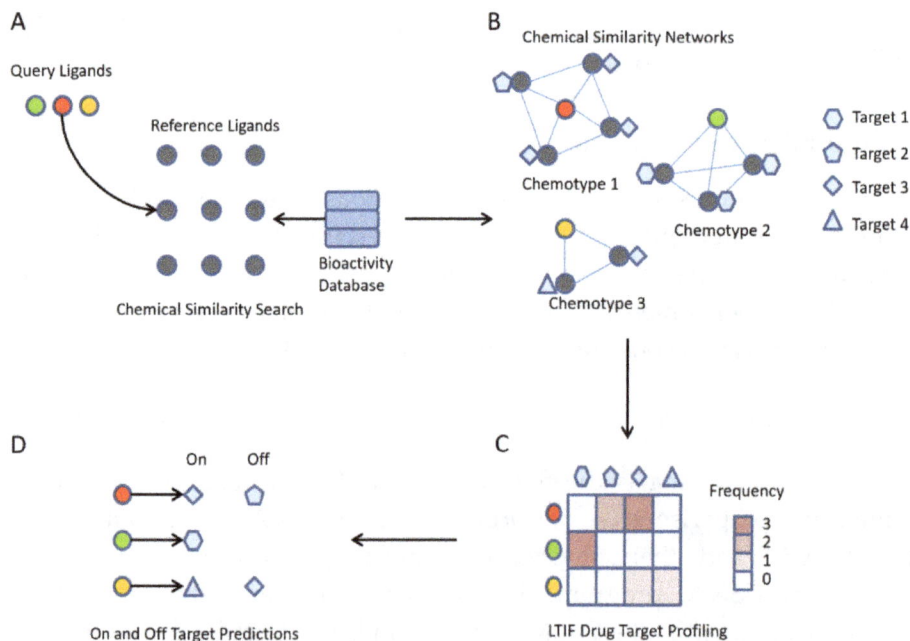

Figure 2. Chemical similarity network analysis pull-down (CSNAP) algorithm for large-scale drug target prediction. (A) Two-dimensional chemical search of three query ligands (green, red, and yellow) identified nine reference compounds from the bioactivity database. (B) Chemical similarity networks clustered compounds into subnetworks corresponding to three major chemotypes. Note that reference compounds interact with four distinct targets. (C) An S-score based on consensus statistics is applied to rank the most probable target based on the target annotation frequency of the first-order neighbor targets. (D) On and off targets are differentiated by ranking the predicted S-scores.

3.2. Case study: CSNAP web server for automated drug target prediction

To reduce concept to practice, we constructed a CSNAP web server for large-scale target prediction and drug discovery. The CSNAP web includes a front-end graphical user interface (GUI) that provides user interaction and output visualization, while target prediction is performed at the back-end by running the CSNAP algorithm.

3.2.1. CSNAP web input

The CSNAP web server accepts two ligand input formats: SDF and SMILES, which are two of the most commonly used molecular formats that handle large compound databases. In addition, a JME molecular editor is also included, which can be used to convert a chemical structure to a SMILES string on the fly (**Figure 3A**). Several chemical fingerprints are provided to perform chemical comparisons during the search and network clustering steps, including Obabel FP2, FP3, PF4, and MACCS fingerprints (**Figure 3B**). Obabel FP2 fingerprints use a path-based algorithm and are more specific than FP3, FP4, and MACCS that utilize a prede-fined set of substructures for chemical searches. On the other hand, when structural analogues are not available in the chemical database, FP3 can instead be used to search structurally distinct chemicals with similar bioactivities. To perform chemical searches, the chemical similarity cutoff needs to be defined. Here, CSNAP web supports a combination of absolute cutoff based on Tanimoto coefficient (Tc > 0.7) and relative chemical similarity cutoff based on a Z-score. From our experience, the default option using a Z-score cutoff of 2.5 will be optimal for most initial CSNAP predictions.

Once the query ligands and chemical search parameters have been defined, the CSNAP algorithm will search the ChEMBL compound activity database to identify structurally similar compounds for target inference (**Figure 3B**). The ChEMBL database assigns targets to a compound based on the level of target specificity (confidence score). Similarly, the compounds are also classified based on the assay type from which they are derived, including biochemical, functional, or ADMET assays. These database parameters will also need to be selected to perform the CSNAP analysis.

3.2.2. CSNAP web output

The CSNAP output page consists of three main panels: (1) chemical similarity networks, (2) chemical structure information, and (3) ligand-target interaction fingerprint (LTIF) (**Figure 3C**).

3.2.3. Chemical similarity networks

The chemical similarity networks panel displays the generated chemical networks using the CSNAP algorithm based on input ligands. The chemical similarity network connects query (red) and annotated ligands (gray) from the ChEMBL database, and the targets are inferred using consensus statistics. For large compound sets, the number of generated chemical clusters can be used to estimate the chemical diversity of the sets. To retrieve additional information regarding a specific ligand, the user can click on the node and the relevant information will be displayed in the chemical structure information panel.

3.2.4. Chemical structure information

The chemical structure information panel displays the chemical information selected from the chemical similarity network panel. The panel consists of several columns that include chemical structure information (chemical ID, chemical structure, SMILES string, InChI key) and the predicted target information (target name and UniProt ID). In the ChEMBL prediction column, the predicted targets of each compound are ranked by the *S*-score.

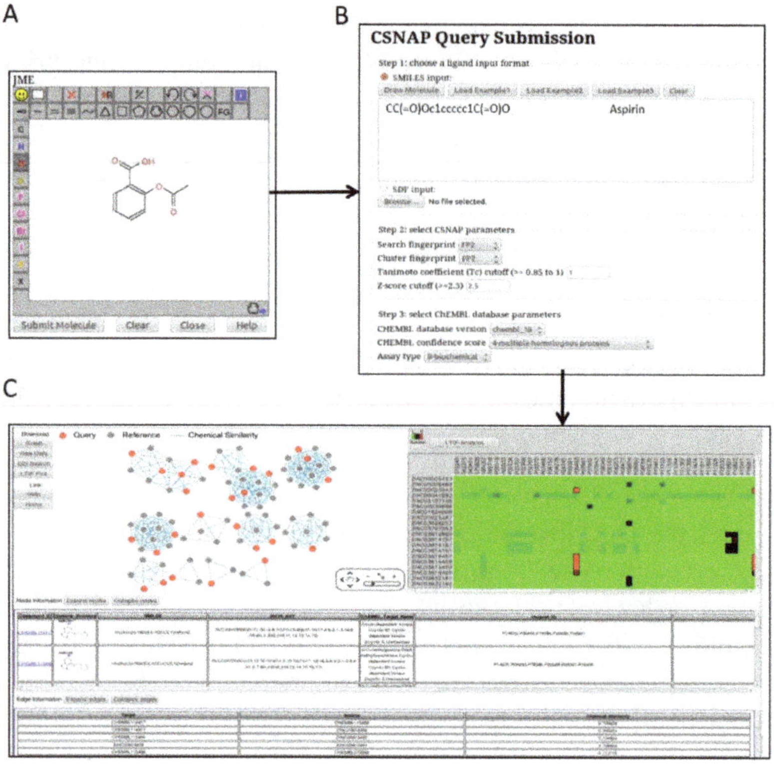

Figure 3. Drug target prediction using the CSNAP web server: (A) construct a query molecule using the JME molecular editor. (B) The molecule is converted to a SMILES string and entered into the CSNAP query submission page. (C) The CSNAP output page consists of three main panels: (1) the chemical similarity network, (2) the chemical structure information, and (3) the ligand-target interaction fingerprint (LTIF).

3.2.5. Ligand-target interaction fingerprint (LTIF)

To analyze the results from large-scale target prediction searches, the ligand-target interaction fingerprint (LTIF) is provided in the CSNAP web output. The LTIF panel displays the predicted *S*-score of each compound mapped against the predicted targets, and the color intensity of the LTIF heatmap is correlated with the *S*-score values. The LTIF can be used to infer compounds sharing similar target binding profiles, which may have similar bioactivity. By clicking on the LTIF button at the top of the LTIF panel, a separate window is created that shows the target spectrum and Gene Ontology (GO) term search derived from the LTIF analysis.

3.2.6. Target spectrum and Gene Ontology (GO) search

To further differentiate primary targets from off-targets in the LTIF, the CSNAP web also computes a target spectrum, by summing the *S*-score ($\sum S$) of all analyzed compounds for each target column (**Figure 4**). For a single compound analysis, the highest peak corresponds to the

primary target. Similarly, for multi-ligand analysis, the highest peak corresponds to the most abundant target in the set. To determine the functional role of the predicted targets, the Gene Ontology (GO) search result is also provided (**Figure 4**). GO is a popular bioinformatics tool that maps genes into functions based on controlled vocabulary (GO terms) and has been widely used for pathway analysis of functional genomic data [20]. Here, CSNAP web incorporates a GO search in target predictions as a strategy for posttarget selection and validation. The GO terms can be used to further select relevant targets in a cell-based or phenotype-based screen based on the knowledge of anticipated molecular etiology including cellular components, molecular functions, and biological process. Smaller subsets of targets can then be filtered for additional experimental validation.

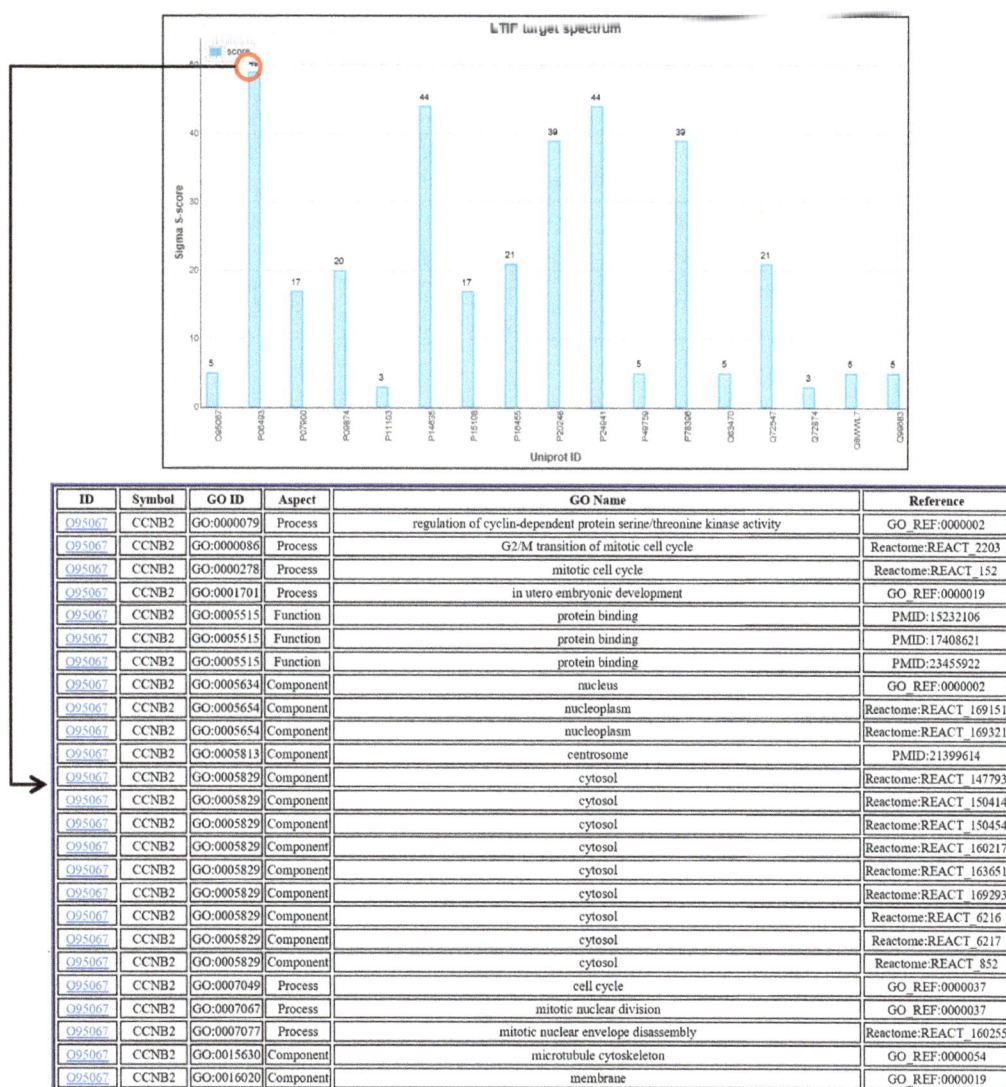

ID	Symbol	GO ID	Aspect	GO Name	Reference
Q95067	CCNB2	GO:0000079	Process	regulation of cyclin-dependent protein serine/threonine kinase activity	GO_REF:0000002
Q95067	CCNB2	GO:0000086	Process	G2/M transition of mitotic cell cycle	Reactome:REACT_2203
Q95067	CCNB2	GO:0000278	Process	mitotic cell cycle	Reactome:REACT_152
Q95067	CCNB2	GO:0001701	Process	in utero embryonic development	GO_REF:0000019
Q95067	CCNB2	GO:0005515	Function	protein binding	PMID:15232106
Q95067	CCNB2	GO:0005515	Function	protein binding	PMID:17408621
Q95067	CCNB2	GO:0005515	Function	protein binding	PMID:23455922
Q95067	CCNB2	GO:0005634	Component	nucleus	GO_REF:0000002
Q95067	CCNB2	GO:0005654	Component	nucleoplasm	Reactome:REACT_169151
Q95067	CCNB2	GO:0005654	Component	nucleoplasm	Reactome:REACT_169321
Q95067	CCNB2	GO:0005813	Component	centrosome	PMID:21399614
Q95067	CCNB2	GO:0005829	Component	cytosol	Reactome:REACT_147793
Q95067	CCNB2	GO:0005829	Component	cytosol	Reactome:REACT_150414
Q95067	CCNB2	GO:0005829	Component	cytosol	Reactome:REACT_150454
Q95067	CCNB2	GO:0005829	Component	cytosol	Reactome:REACT_160217
Q95067	CCNB2	GO:0005829	Component	cytosol	Reactome:REACT_163651
Q95067	CCNB2	GO:0005829	Component	cytosol	Reactome:REACT_169293
Q95067	CCNB2	GO:0005829	Component	cytosol	Reactome:REACT_6216
Q95067	CCNB2	GO:0005829	Component	cytosol	Reactome:REACT_6217
Q95067	CCNB2	GO:0005829	Component	cytosol	Reactome:REACT_852
Q95067	CCNB2	GO:0007049	Process	cell cycle	GO_REF:0000037
Q95067	CCNB2	GO:0007067	Process	mitotic nuclear division	GO_REF:0000037
Q95067	CCNB2	GO:0007077	Process	mitotic nuclear envelope disassembly	Reactome:REACT_160255
Q95067	CCNB2	GO:0015630	Component	microtubule cytoskeleton	GO_REF:0000054
Q95067	CCNB2	GO:0016020	Component	membrane	GO_REF:0000019

Figure 4. Posttarget validation using Gene Ontology (GO) analysis in the CSNAP web. (Top) Target spectrum. (Bottom) GO search results.

4. Application of CSNAP for drug target prediction and discovery

4.1. CSNAP validation

The CSNAP algorithm was validated using 206 known drugs from the directory of useful decoy (DUD) set [21]. The benchmark set included 46 angiotensin-converting enzyme (ACE), 47 cyclin-dependent kinase 2 (CDK2), 23 heat-shock protein 90 (HSP90), 34 HIV reverse-transcriptase (HIVRT), 25 HMG-CoA reductase (HMGA), and 31 poly [ADP-ribose] polymerase (PARP) inhibitors. Using the default search criteria (fingerprint: FP2, Tc = 1, Z-score = 2.5), we evaluated the ability of the CSNAP algorithm to accurately predict the designated targets of each compound based on the S-score rankings. CSNAP analysis of the 206 compounds showed that the chemical similarity network clustered the drugs into distinct subnetworks, corresponding to diverse chemical scaffolds (chemotypes) (**Figure 5**). For a given subnetwork, the S-score was further used to predict the drug target of each compound based on their network connectivity with the reference ligands. The prediction results were then compared with those obtained by the similarity ensemble approach (SEA) [22]. The CSNAP algorithm gave an overall 80–94% true-positive prediction rate (TPR) in comparison with SEA (63–75%) based on the top 1, top 5, and top 10 ranking of target predictions. In particular, CSNAP substantially improved the target prediction rate for promiscuous ligands such as CDK2 and ACE inhibitors (92 and 96%) compared to the SEA approach (30 and 65%) (**Figure 6**).

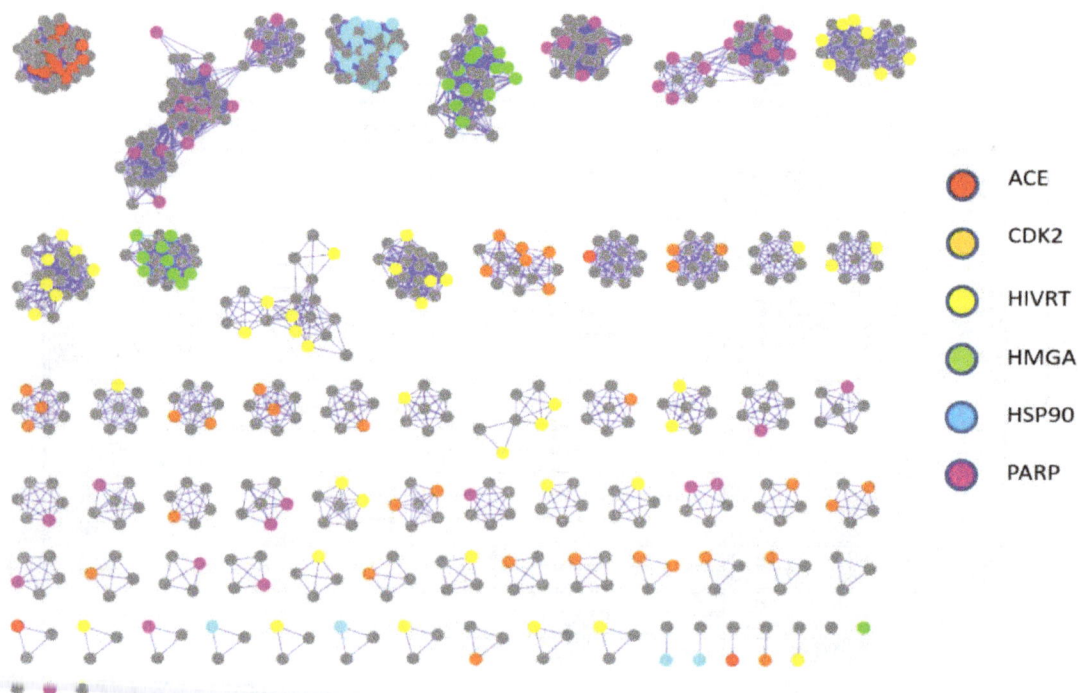

Figure 5. CSNAP2D clustering of 206 benchmark compounds consisting of six known drug classes from the directory of useful decoy (DUD) set.

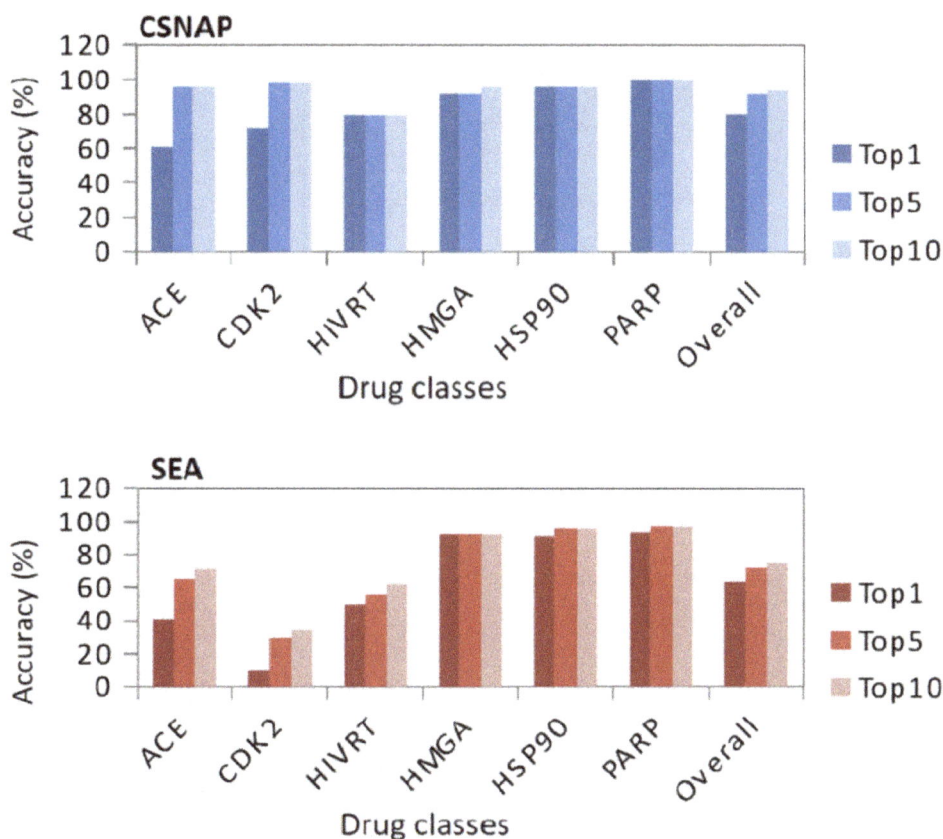

Figure 6. Performance comparison between CSNAP and SEA. CSNAP achieved improved prediction accuracy (TPR) for promiscuous drug classes like ACE, CDK2, and HIVRT inhibitors.

4.2. Target prediction of hits from an antimitotic chemical screen

We applied the CSNAP algorithm to predict the drug targets of a set of 212 compounds that were inhibitors of cell division [23]. CSNAP clustering of the mitotic compounds resulted into 85 chemical similarity subnetworks (**Figure 7A**). To identify the most common targets within the set, we applied the LTIF analysis. The target spectrum derived from the LTIF revealed four broad classes of mitotic targets including fatty acid desaturases (SCD, SCD1, and FADS2), ABL1 kinase, non-receptor-type tyrosine phosphatases (PTPN7, PTPN12, PTPN22, PTPRC, and ACP1), and beta tubulins. In particular, the target spectrum showed that beta tubulin had the largest peak height and was the most prominent protein target for the mitotic compounds. Further analysis showed that 51 compounds were associated with tubulin-targeting chemo-types. The predicted drug targets were validated by comparing siRNA-treated and drug-treated mitotic phenotypes in cell culture using immunofluorescence microscopy. In addition, *in vitro* tubulin polymerization assays were used to determine the effects of these compounds on microtubule formation. Among the 51 tested compounds, 31 compounds showed a perturbation of microtubule polymerization >25%, and thus, the CSNAP algorithm achieved a prediction accuracy of >70%.

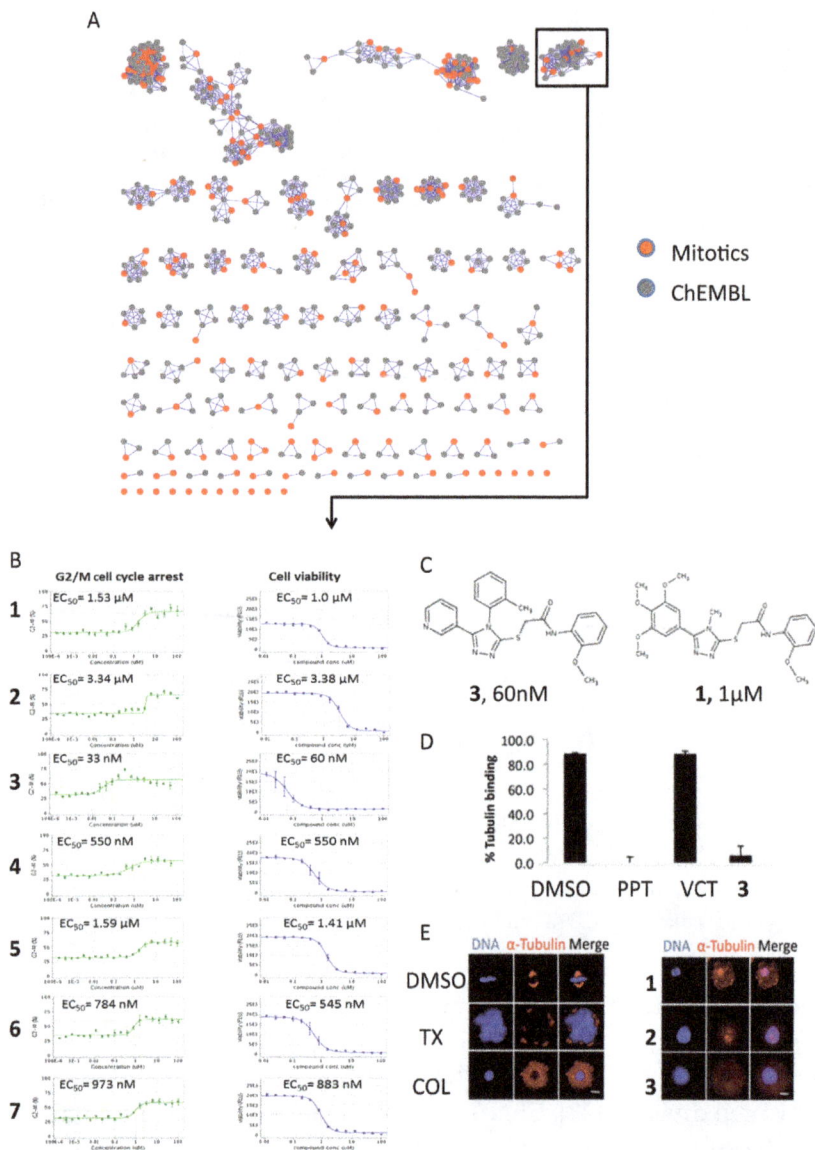

Figure 7. Discovery of novel tubulin-targeting drugs (compounds **1–7**). (A) CSNAP analysis of 212 mitotic drugs identified seven novel tubulin destabilizing compounds. (B) The compounds induced a G2/M cell cycle arrest and decreased cell viability in cell-based assays. (C) Discovery of compound **3** as the most potent compound in the series. (D) A mass spectrometry-based competition assay was used to show that compound **3** and podophyllotoxin (PPT) competed for binding to tubulin in contrast to vincristine (VCT). (E) Compound-treated (**1–3**) and colchicine-treated (COL) cells displayed a tubulin destabilizing effect in comparison with the tubulin stabilizing effect of taxol (TX).

4.3. Discovery of novel tubulin-targeting antimitotics

Using a negative selection strategy, we identified seven novel tubulin-targeting agents that were active in our tubulin polymerization assay but had not been associated with known tubulin chemotypes (**Figure 7A**). The seven compounds were analogues of phenyl-sulfanyl-thiazol-acetamide scaffolds that exhibit various degrees of tubulin destabilizing effects through a mechanism similar to that of the tubulin destabilizing agent colchicine. The most potent compound, compound **3**, in the series exhibited a cytotoxic effect in the nano-molar range (EC_{50}: G2/M = 33 nM; EC_{50}: cell death = 60 nM) when evaluated in cell viability and G2/M arrest assays (**Figure 7B, C**) [15]. The predicted mechanism was validated using a mass spectrometry-based competition assay where both the selected analogues and podophyllotoxin, a known colchicine site binder, competed for binding to tubulin in contrast to the negative control vincristine that interacted with a distant site in beta tubulin (**Figure 7D**) [24]. Likewise, both compound-treated and colchicine-treated cells displayed a tubulin destabilizing phenotype, characterized by rapid shortening of microtubule length and the disappearance of microtubule polymer mass (**Figure 7E**).

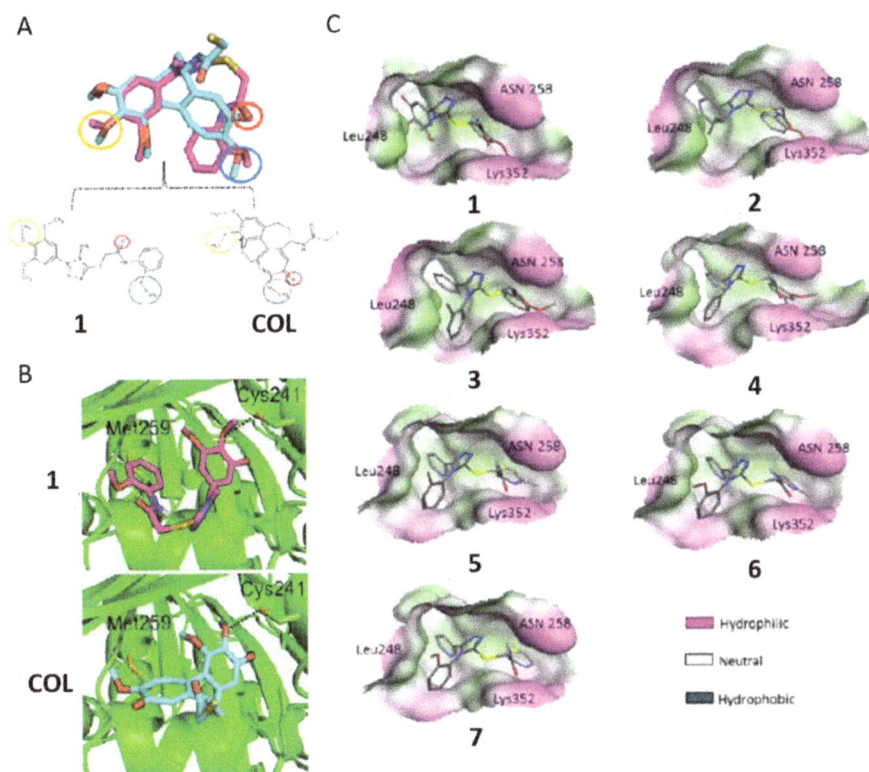

Figure 8. Binding mechanism of a novel tubulin destabilizing chemotype (compounds **1–7**). (A) Pharmacophore alignment between compound **1** and colchicine (COL) showed a consensus pharmacophore. (B) Docking of compound **1** in the colchicine site using the tubulin crystal structure (PDB code: 1SA0) revealed colchicine-like interactions with critical residues (Met259, Cys241). (C) Docking of the seven analogues into the colchicine site showed similar interactions.

4.4. Characterization of novel tubulin-targeting antimitotics

To investigate how the novel antimitotics interacted with beta tubulin, we performed structural alignments between compound **6** and colchicine and identified a consensus pharmacophore between the two molecules (**Figure 8A**). Further docking of compound **6** into the colchicine binding site also showed that both compound **6** and colchicine interacted with common residues, including the 2 and 10 methoxy groups and 9-keto group that interacted with Met259 and Cys241 of beta tubulin, respectively (**Figure 8B**). Similarly, all seven analogues docked into the same site through similar interactions. Interestingly, the elucidated binding modes could be used to explain the observed SAR. For example, the increased potency of compound **7** and **8** in comparison with **6** could be attributed to the hydrophilic interactions between the *N*-propyl and *N*-phenyl groups with Leu248 and Lys352 within the subpockets of the colchicine binding site (**Figure 8C**).

5. CSNAP3D: a 3D upgrade to the CSNAP approach

Chemical similarity searches based on 2D chemical structures have several limitations. First, compounds with distinct scaffolds can exhibit similar bioactivity due to "scaffold hopping" by interacting with a common receptor [25, 26]. Second, although 2D fingerprints based on substructure or fragment searches have the potential to detect scaffold hopping, the scaffold enrichment rate is low. Furthermore, 2D searches do not capture essential features of protein-ligand interactions in three-dimensional space. Consequently, 3D chemical searches based on the three-dimensional information of the ligands will offer additional opportunities to discover novel compounds.

5.1. 3D chemical similarity search

The most common approach to compare ligand similarity in 3D is by shape superposition, which maximizes the Gaussian volume overlap between two ligands [27]. Alternatively, ligand alignments that use molecular interaction field (MIF) or pharmacophore have also been proposed [28, 29]. These approaches take into account the shared chemical features arranged in three-dimensional space. To identify the optimal 3D chemical descriptors, we performed an unbiased screen of diverse 3D chemical descriptors based on molecular shapes or pharmacophores. Using 206 benchmark compounds from the DUD set, we tested the ability of each 3D descriptor to enrich class-specific scaffolds ranked by respective similarity scores. The lowest energy conformer of each ligand was generated using the MOE program. The results showed that 3D chemical descriptors using a combination of shape and pharmacophore features achieved the highest enrichment rate and ligand alignment accuracy compared to those based on shape or pharmacophore alone. This observation agrees with our current understanding that shape complementary and chemical matching are essential for the protein-ligand binding process.

We subsequently developed a 3D chemical similarity search method called "ShapeAlign" that utilized two open-source softwares: "Shape-it" and "Align-it" [30]. Similar to the combo score implemented in the ROCS program, the ShapeAlign algorithm also used a combination of shape and pharmacophore for 3D chemical searches. However, ShapeAlign incorporated a 2D fingerprint similarity score as an integral part of the searching process. Given a ligand with a pre-generated 3D conformation, the ShapeAlign algorithm first detects ligands from the chemical database with the highest shape matching evaluated by a shape Tanimoto index. The hit molecules are then aligned and rescored according to the degree of pharmacophore matching using the Align-it program.

5.2. Drug target prediction using CSNAP3D

We incorporated the "ShapeAlign" algorithm into our CSNAP program called "CSNAP3D" to cluster chemical structures and predict drug targets based on 3D ligand similarity. To evaluate CSNAP3D performance, we assessed the average true-positive rate (TPR) and false-positive rate (FPR) of predicting drug targets for the 206 benchmark compounds. The result showed that CSNAP3D achieved a TPR of >95% at 0.85 Tanimoto cutoff in comparison with other 2D target prediction approaches including CSNAP2D, SEA, and PASS approaches [17]. A comparison of CSNAP3D and CSNAP2D generated networks showed that diverse 2D scaffold subnetworks were clustered into smaller subsets of 3D chemical networks, suggesting that CSNAP3D could be used to identify scaffold hopping ligands not identifiable by conventional 2D methods (**Figure 9**).

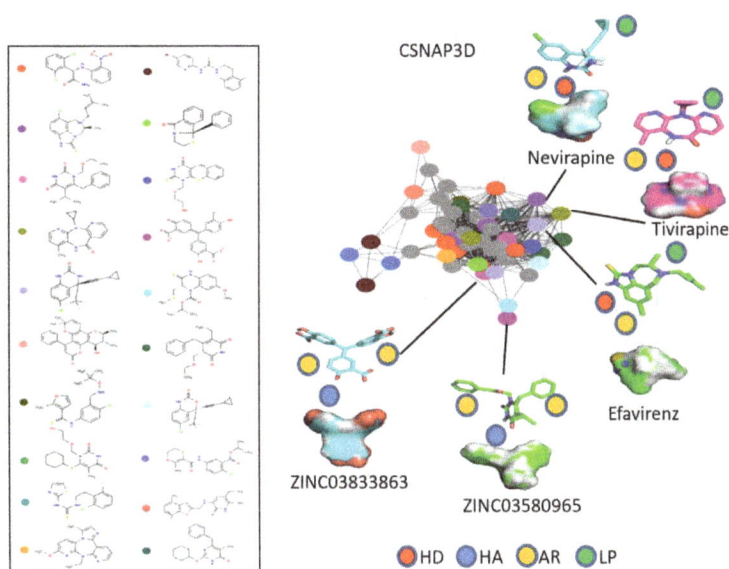

Figure 9. CSNAP3D clustered 34 distinct HIVRT NNRTI chemotypes into a shape-based chemical similarity network. The figure shows that many NNRTIs are scaffold hopping ligands to a common nucleotidyltransferase binding site. The 3D alignment between ligands was based on molecular shape and pharmacophore points (HD: hydrogen donor, HA: hydrogen acceptor, AR: aromatic, LP: lipophilic).

5.2.1. Target prediction of HIVRT inhibitors

As further validation, we presented a case study of predicting targets for a set of HIVRT inhibitors using the CSNAP3D algorithm. HIVRT inhibitors can be classified as nucleoside-based analogues (NRTIs) or non-nucleoside-based analogues (NNRTIs) [31]. In particular, NNRTIs have been difficult drug classes for computational dug target prediction due to the chemical diversity of the drug classes where many compounds are scaffold hopping ligands that bind to a common nucleotidyltransferase binding site. Although 3D ligand-based target predictions that use either the alignment or nonalignment methods have been attempted, many of these approaches yielded low predictability. Here, we applied CSNAP3D to predict the drug targets of 34 structurally diverse HIVRT NNRTIs and compared the prediction results with the CSNAP2D approach (**Figure 9**). Initial 2D chemical similarity network analysis clustered the 34 NNRTIs into 20 structurally diverse chemical similarity scaffolds. Further LTIF analysis, by mapping target prediction S-scores to the heatmap, showed that more than 20 compounds did not have a prediction. The NNRTIs were similarly analyzed by the CSNAP3D program using the ShapeAlign algorithm. In contrast, all the 34 ligands were clustered by CSNAP3D into a single shape-based chemical similarity network, suggesting that many NNRTIs are scaffold hopping ligands to a common binding site. LTIF analysis showed that 33 of NNRTIs were correctly predicted, thus achieving a TPR of >97%. In particular, 3D chemical similarity networks correctly identify three FDA-approved NNRTIs, namely efavirenz, nevirapine, and tivirapine whose structure alignment agreed with previous crystal structures and SAR studies (**Figure 9**). In addition, several novel scaffold hopping pairs were also identified (**Figure 9**).

5.2.2. Discovery of novel taxol scaffold hopping ligands

Taxol (paclitaxel) is a well-known anticancer natural product derived from the Yew tree, whose antiproliferative effect was first discovered in 1960s from an NCI anticancer drug screening campaign [32]. Taxol has since been found to be effective for treating a wide range of cancers including ovarian, breast, lung, bladder, prostate, melanoma, esophageal, and other solid tumors. However, the efficacy of taxol has been limited by severe side effects, toxicity, and synthetic feasibility. Thus, identification of low-weight taxol mimetics with more tolerable drug profiles is critical. While several taxol mimetics have been discovered including Synstab B and GS-164, both discovered by chemical screening, their binding mechanisms have remained undetermined [33, 34].

Here, we sought a rational approach to discover taxol mimetics using the CSNAP3D algorithm based on our existing structural knowledge of the original taxol molecule. CSNAP3D analysis of the 212 mitotic compounds from a chemical screen identified 42 potential taxol mimetics linked to 30 taxol structural conformers. Seven predicted taxol mimetics were found to be true positives with a >25% fold change in optical density when tested in tubulin polymerization assays *in vitro* and four compounds shared a consensus chemotype by co-localizing within one chemical similarity subnetwork. The structural alignment of the four selected molecules with taxol showed that they shared a similar T-shape conformation despite a simpler scaffold (**Figure 10A**). Docking studies showed that the increase in microtubule polymerization activity could be attributed to the phenyl moiety of these ligands, which was capable of forming a pi–pi stacking interaction with the critical residue His229 within the taxane site (**Figure 10B**). Three of the compounds demonstrated cytotoxic and antimitotic effects in cell culture with a potency <5 µM. Similarly, all the compounds displayed a similar tubulin stabilizing phenotype, characterized by microtubule aster formation in immunofluorescence microscopy studies (**Figure 10C**).

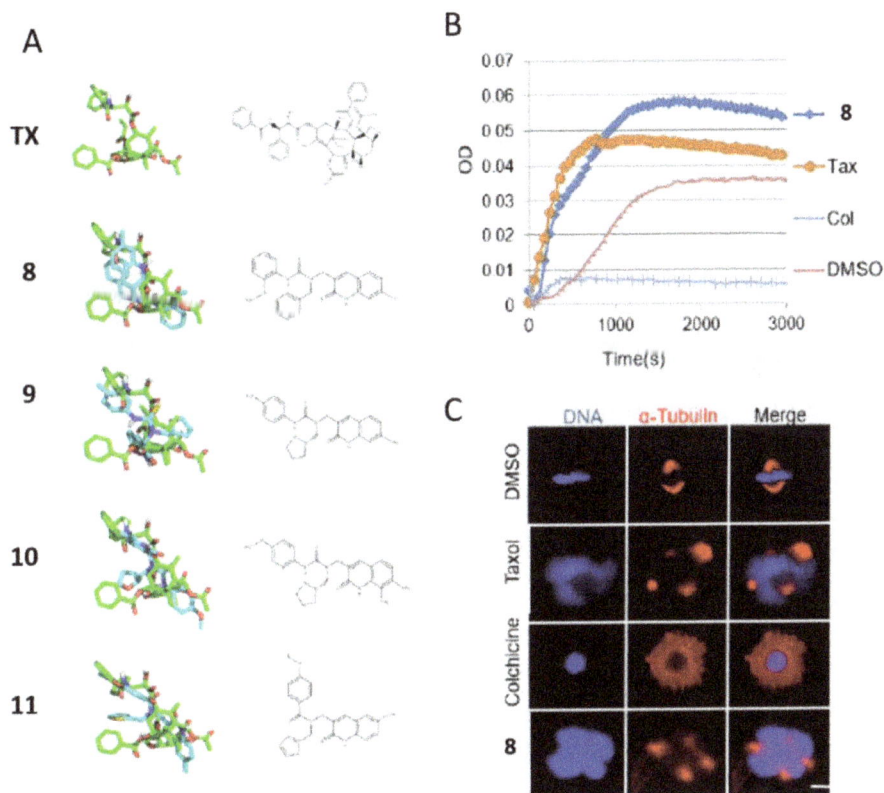

Figure 10. Structure-based discovery of taxol mimetics. (A) CSNAP3D analysis of 212 mitotic compounds from a cell-based screen identified four low molecular weight taxol (TX) mimetic analogues. (B) Compound **8 (8)** demonstrated a fast tubulin polymerization rate at 50 μM similar to taxol (Tax) at 5 μM in comparison with colchicine (Col). (C) Compound **8** displayed a tubulin stabilizing phenotype, characterized by microtubule aster formation in immunofluorescence microscopy studies.

6. Conclusions and future directions

Chemical similarity is an important concept in medicinal chemistry and drug discovery to identify similar compounds with improved bioactivities. Here, we have expanded on this concept to chemical similarity network theory, where descriptive network statistics and graph topology can be applied to large-scale analysis of chemical diversity, bioactivities, and target identification. To demonstrate the utility of this approach, we have implemented the CSNAP algorithm, which can be used for large-scale compound analysis and target predictions. Analogous to protein function prediction in PPI networks, we applied consensus statistics to identify the common targets of each query ligand. We showed that this scoring function outperforms several target prediction methods based on simple chemical similarity searches. To address the challenge of scaffold hopping, where structurally diverse ligands can potentially interact with a common receptor, we developed the CSNAP3D algorithm as a CSNAP extension. CSNAP3D searches chemical structure using the "ShapeAlign" protocol, which utilizes a combination of shape and pharmacophore descriptors. We found that CSNAP3D improves target prediction, particularly for challenging drug classes such as HIVRT NNRTIs that showed high structural diversity and are scaffold hopping ligands. Finally, we successfully applied CSNAP3D to rationally discover low molecular weight taxol mimetics, which exhibit a taxol-like anticancer mechanism and potentially possess improved transport and pharmacokinetic properties than its natural counterpart.

The current CSNAP framework can be extended in several directions. For instance, consensus scoring can be expanded by considering higher-order neighbors, which has been demonstrated to improve prediction accuracy in PPI networks. Similarly, graph theoretical approaches based on maximum network flow and other global optimization approaches can be applied for target assignments [35]. To improve posttarget validation, high throughput functional genomics data can be incorporated to aid in the identification of critical targets relevant to a disease pathway. One example is multiplayer network approaches that integrate drug, target, and annotation interaction networks to enhance target predictions and validations [36]. While CSNAP3D has substantially improved the predictability of CSNAP2D, the algorithm is limited to receptors with bound ligands and the ligand alignment is based on the lowest energy conformer. This shortcoming can be circumvented by considering multi-conformer networks that correlate ligand conformation with target specificities. Likewise, pseudo-ligands generated as the mirror image of an orphan receptor can be considered for receptor deorphanization.

In conclusion, chemical similarity networks are an emerging field in ligand-based drug discovery where the collective properties of a ligand can be easily dissected using descriptive network statistics and graph topology. Here, we presented a new network-based approach for drug discovery and target identification called chemical similarity network analysis pull-down (CSNAP) and a new CSNAP framework called CSNAP3D. The CSNAP computational framework represents a new concept in computational drug discovery with practical application in target identification and drug discovery. We anticipate that the CSNAP approach will stimulate further work in systems and network-based drug discovery that will aid in the discovery of novel drugs for the treatment of cancer and other important diseases.

Author details

Yu-Chen Lo[1] and Jorge Z. Torres[2*]

*Address all correspondence to: torres@chem.ucla.edu

1 Department of Bioengineering, Stanford University, Stanford, CA, USA

2 Department of Chemistry and Biochemistry, University of California, Los Angeles, CA, USA

References

[1] Yan X, Liao C, Liu Z, Hagler AT, Gu Q, Xu J. Chemical structure similarity search for ligand-based virtual screening: methods and computational resources. Current Drug Targets. 2015, Vol. 16, 1p.

[2] Willett P. Chemoinformatics—similarity and diversity in chemical libraries. Current Opinion in Biotechnology. 2000;11(1):85–8.

[3] Maggiora G, Vogt M, Stumpfe D, Bajorath J. Molecular similarity in medicinal chemistry. Journal of Medicinal Chemistry. 2014;57(8):3186–204.

[4] Faulon J-L, Bender A. Handbook of chemoinformatics algorithms. Boca Raton, FL: Chapman & Hall/CRC; 2010. xii, 440 p.

[5] Gasteiger J. Handbook of chemoinformatics: from data to knowledge. Weinheim: Wiley-VCH; 2003.

[6] Lee JK. Statistical bioinformatics: a guide for life and biomedical science researchers. Hoboken, NJ: Wiley-Blackwell; 2010. xiv, 350 p., 20 p. of plates p.

[7] Baldi P, Benz RW. BLASTing small molecules--statistics and extreme statistics of chemical similarity scores. Bioinformatics. 2008;24(13):i357–65.

[8] Consonni V, Todeschini R, Pavan M, Gramatica P. Structure/response correlations and similarity/diversity analysis by GETAWAY descriptors. 2. Application of the novel 3D molecular descriptors to QSAR/QSPR studies. Journal of Chemical Information and Computer Science. 2002;42(3):693–705.

[9] Devinyak O, Havrylyuk D, Lesyk R. 3D-MoRSE descriptors explained. Journal of Molecular Graphics and Modelling. 2014;54:194–203.

[10] Hopkins AL. Network pharmacology. Nature Biotechnology. 2007;25(10):1110–1.

[11] Lounkine E, Keiser MJ, Whitebread S, Mikhailov D, Hamon J, Jenkins JL, et al. Large-scale prediction and testing of drug activity on side-effect targets. Nature. 2012;486(7403):361–7.

[12] Gaulton A, Bellis LJ, Bento AP, Chambers J, Davies M, Hersey A, et al. ChEMBL: a large-scale bioactivity database for drug discovery. Nucleic Acids Research. 2012;40(Database issue):D1100–7.

[13] Li Q, Cheng T, Wang Y, Bryant SH. PubChem as a public resource for drug discovery. Drug Discovery Today. 2010;15(23–24):1052–7.

[14] Wishart DS, Knox C, Guo AC, Shrivastava S, Hassanali M, Stothard P, et al. DrugBank: a comprehensive resource for in silico drug discovery and exploration. Nucleic Acids Research. 2006;34(Database issue):D668–72.

[15] Lo YC, Senese S, Li CM, Hu Q, Huang Y, Damoiseaux R, et al. Large-scale chemical similarity networks for target profiling of compounds identified in cell-based chemical screens. PLoS Computational Biology. 2015;11(3):e1004153.

[16] Schwikowski B, Uetz P, Fields S. A network of protein-protein interactions in yeast. Nature Biotechnology. 2000;18(12):1257–61.

[17] Lo YC, Senese S, Damoiseaux R, Torres JZ. 3D chemical similarity networks for structure-based target prediction and Scaffold hopping. ACS Chemical Biology. 2016;11(8):2244–53.

[18] Aretz I, Meierhofer D. Advantages and pitfalls of mass spectrometry based metabolome profiling in systems biology. International Journal of Molecular Sciences. 2016;17:632.

[19] Kolaczyk ED. Statistical analysis of network data: methods and models. New York; London: Springer; 2009. xii, 386 p.

[20] Ashburner M, Ball CA, Blake JA, Botstein D, Butler H, Cherry JM, et al. Gene ontology: tool for the unification of biology. The Gene Ontology Consortium. Nature Genetics. 2000;25(1):25–9.

[21] Mysinger MM, Carchia M, Irwin JJ, Shoichet BK. Directory of useful decoys, enhanced (DUD-E): better ligands and decoys for better benchmarking. Journal of Medicinal Chemistry. 2012;55(14):6582–94.

[22] Keiser MJ, Roth BL, Armbruster BN, Ernsberger P, Irwin JJ, Shoichet BK. Relating protein pharmacology by ligand chemistry. Nature Biotechnology. 2007;25(2):197–206.

[23] Senese S, Lo YC, Huang D, Zangle TA, Gholkar AA, Robert L, et al. Chemical dissection of the cell cycle: probes for cell biology and anti-cancer drug development. Cell Death & Disease. 2014;5:e1462.

[24] Li CM, Lu Y, Ahn S, Narayanan R, Miller DD, Dalton JT. Competitive mass spectrometry binding assay for characterization of three binding sites of tubulin. Journal of Mass Spectrometry. 2010;45(10):1160–6.

[25] Schneider G, Neidhart W, Giller T, Schmid G. "Scaffold-Hopping" by topological pharmacophore search: a contribution to virtual screening. Angewandte Chemie, International Edition in English. 1999;38(19):2894–6.

[26] Sun H, Tawa G, Wallqvist A. Classification of scaffold-hopping approaches. Drug Discovery Today. 2012;17(7–8):310–24.

[27] Yan X, Li J, Liu Z, Zheng M, Ge H, Xu J. Enhancing molecular shape comparison by weighted Gaussian functions. Journal of Chemical Information and Modeling. 2013;53(8):1967–78.

[28] Cruciani G. Molecular interaction fields: applications in drug discovery and ADME prediction. Weinheim: Wiley-VCH; 2006. xviii, 307 p.

[29] Liu X, Ouyang S, Yu B, Liu Y, Huang K, Gong J, et al. PharmMapper server: a web server for potential drug target identification using pharmacophore mapping approach. Nucleic Acids Research. 2010;38(Web Server issue):W609–14.

[30] Taminau J, Thijs G, De Winter H. Pharao: pharmacophore alignment and optimization. Journal of Molecular Graphics and Modelling. 2008;27(2):161–9.

[31] Zhan P, Chen X, Li D, Fang Z, De Clercq E, Liu X. HIV-1 NNRTIs: structural diversity, pharmacophore similarity, and implications for drug design. Medicinal Research Reviews. 2013;33(Suppl 1):E1–72.

[32] Renneberg R. Biotech History: Yew trees, paclitaxel synthesis and fungi. Biotechnology Journal. 2007;2(10):1207–9.

[33] Haggarty SJ, Mayer TU, Miyamoto DT, Fathi R, King RW, Mitchison TJ, et al. Dissecting cellular processes using small molecules: identification of colchicine-like, taxol-like and other small molecules that perturb mitosis. Chemistry & Biology. 2000;7(4):275–86.

[34] Shintani Y, Tanaka T, Nozaki Y. GS-164, a small synthetic compound, stimulates tubulin polymerization by a similar mechanism to that of taxol. Cancer Chemotherapy and Pharmacology. 1997;40(6):513–20.

[35] Jungnickel D. Graphs, networks, and algorithms. Fourth edition. ed. Heidelberg; New York: Springer; 2013. xx, 675 p.

[36] Berenstein AJ, Magarinos MP, Chernomoretz A, Aguero F. A multilayer network approach for guiding drug repositioning in neglected diseases. PLoS Neglected Tropical Diseases. 2016;10(1):e0004300.

3

Autobioluminescent Cellular Models for Enhanced Drug Discovery

Tingting Xu, Michael Conway, Ashley Frank,
Amelia Brumbaugh, Steven Ripp and Dan Close

Additional information is available at the end of the chapter

Abstract

Autobioluminescent cellular models are emerging tools for drug discovery that rely on the expression of a synthetic, eukaryotic-optimized luciferase that does not require an exogenous chemical substrate to produce its resultant output signal. These models can therefore self-modulate their output signals in response to metabolic activity dynamics and avoid the sample destruction and intermittent data acquisition limitations of traditional fluorescent or chemically stimulated bioluminescent approaches. While promising for reducing drug discovery costs and increasing data acquisition relative to alternative approaches, these models have remained relatively untested for drug discovery applications due to their recent emergence within the field. This chapter presents a history and background of these autobioluminescent cellular models to offer investigators a generalized point of reference for understanding their capabilities and limitations and provides side-by-side comparisons between autobioluminescent and traditional, substrate-requiring toxicology screening platforms for pharmaceutically relevant three-dimensional and high-throughput screening applications to introduce investigators to autobioluminescence as a potential new drug discovery toolset.

Keywords: luciferase, *lux*, toxicology, high-throughput screening, three-dimensional cell culture, drug discovery

1. Introduction to autobioluminescence

1.1. A brief overview of autobioluminescence

Autobioluminescence is defined as the ability of a cell to self-initiate the production of a luminescent signal using only endogenously supplied substrates to perform the enzymatic reactions necessary for signal generation. In this regard, it is separate from traditional bioluminescence in that it is not dependent on the exogenous addition of a chemical substrate to supplement the metabolic cosubstrates that are naturally present within cells expressing an associated luciferase protein. Interestingly, under this definition, there are many examples of autobioluminescence in nature that can be found across a diverse array of organisms such as bacteria, dinoflagellates, fungi, and beetles [1]. However, of these natural autobioluminescent systems, only that of the bacteria (commonly referred to as the *lux* system) has been successfully transitioned as a reporter system for scientific applications while maintaining its autonomous functionality [2–4]. The remaining systems, such as firefly luciferase, *Renilla* luciferase, and *Gaussia* luciferase, have been limited in this transition by incomplete understandings of the genetic frameworks behind their substrate production biochemical pathways or limitations on the abilities of host cells to support the endogenous production of all the components required for their expression. These systems therefore all require the external application of a chemical substrate (D-luciferin for firefly luciferase and coelenterazine for *Renilla* and *Gaussia* luciferase) to activate their light production under scientifically relevant applications [5].

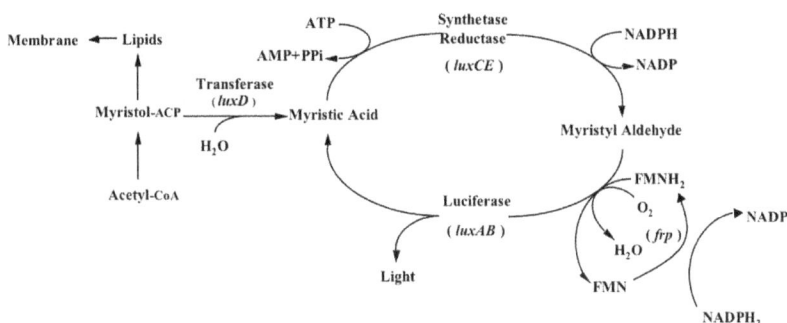

Figure 1. The autobioluminescent reaction catalyzed by the bacterial luciferase gene cassette. The luciferase is formed from a heterodimer of the *luxA* and *luxB* gene products. The aliphatic aldehyde is supplied and regenerated by the products of the *luxC*, *luxD*, and *luxE* genes. The required oxygen and reduced riboflavin phosphate substrates are scavenged from endogenous metabolic processes and the flavin reductase gene (*frp*) aids in reduced flavin turnover rates in some species. Used with permission from [7] under a Creative Commons Attribution-Noncommercial license.

The successfully transitioned bacterial *lux* system, alternatively, utilizes a characterized core set of five genes, *luxC*, *luxD*, *luxA*, *luxB*, and *luxE*, to express both its luciferase enzyme (a dimer formed by the *luxA* and *luxB* gene products) and its supporting transferase (*luxD*), reductase (*luxC*), and synthetase (*luxE*) enzymes that supply the required aldehyde substrate from natural cellular metabolic components. In addition, this reaction also requires the metabolites $FMNH_2$ and O_2 in order to function, producing a luminescent output at 490 nm and a reduced corresponding acid compound, FMN, and H_2O as products [6] (**Figure 1**). Interestingly, despite the relatively straightforward organization of this system and the longstanding elucidation of its individual components roles and genetic identities, there were significant hurdles that needed to be overcome before it could be successfully transitioned for expression in the mammalian systems that are required for drug discovery applications.

1.2. History of autobioluminescent cellular model development

Due to its bacterial origin, the *lux* cassette was formerly believed to function solely in prokaryotic hosts, and thus was not considered a viable tool for diagnostic screening in human cell lines [8]. This belief was due to the initial difficulty researchers encountered in coordinating the temporal and spatial coexpression of the multiple *lux* genes, the thermoinstability of the *lux* proteins at the mammalian optimal temperature of 37°C, and the limited availability of the $FMNH_2$ cosubstrate within human cells relative to their uncompartmentalized bacterial counterparts. As a result of these initial difficulties, alternative bioluminescent systems became more popular for use in drug discovery applications. In particular, firefly luciferase (*luc*) has become the dominant bioluminescent imaging target for this application due to its single gene expression requirement, high quantum yield, and favorable output signal wavelength of 562 nm [9].

However, despite the initial challenges associated with transitioning the bacterial *lux* system into mammalian cells, significant progress was made over the years that would eventually lead to the development of an optimized version of the system that could function reliably within the human cellular microenvironment. The first major stepping stone in this process was the expression of a functional luciferase heterodimer (*luxAB*) in the human kidney cell line HEK293 by Patterson et al. in 2005 [10]. This demonstration was particularly important because Patterson and her colleagues were able to overcome the previous limitations of both spatial/temporal coexpression and protein thermostability. Unlike previous work that had attempted to coordinately express the genes using short protein linker sequences or individual promoters [11–16], Patterson et al. linked the *luxA* and *luxB* genes using an internal ribosomal entry site (IRES) element to allow for expression of individual protein products from a single mRNA transcript. Thermostability issues were overcome by using human codon optimized gene sequences corresponding to the less utilized *Photorhabdus luminescens* bacterial system, which allowed for higher levels of transgene expression of proteins with greater thermal tolerance than those of the traditionally employed *Aliivibrio fischeri* (previously *Vibrio fischeri*) system [17].

Further advances were made to the *lux* system by Close et al. in 2010 that built heavily upon the techniques developed by Patterson et al. [18]. This later work expanded the earlier IRES-based expression strategy to coexpress pairs of *lux* genes from individual promoters and divide the expression of the genes across two plasmids. Most importantly, however, Close and his colleagues were able to overcome the limitation of signal output strength imparted by the low level of endogenously available $FMNH_2$ by including a sixth gene (*frp*) that encoded for a flavin reductase enzyme. This enzyme was able to rapidly recycle the oxidized FMN in the mammalian cytosol into $FMNH_2$, which increased light output to the point where it could be visualized externally using commonly available detection equipment. This marked the first demonstration of autobioluminescence in a host system amenable to drug discovery applications, however, the autobioluminescent output levels from this approach were significantly lower than traditional bioluminescent systems and the use of multiple plasmids and large, repetitive IRES element DNA sequences made the system difficult to work with on a molecular biology level.

These difficulties were later overcome by Xu et al. in 2014, who re-optimized the system for expression from a single promoter and therefore allowed it to be expressed from a single plasmid [19]. This approach, which substituted viral 2A elements in place of the previously employed IRES elements, allowed the full autobioluminescent DNA cassette to be manipulated as a single gene and significantly increased the signal output level to the point where it could be detected from the low numbers of cells that are commonly used in high throughput screening applications. Using the new expression format, Xu and her colleagues were able to demonstrate the use of autobioluminescent reporters for tracking cellular metabolic dynamics, population sizes, and promoter activation events, finally demonstrating the use of autobioluminescence for the same applications as traditional bioluminescent reporter systems [19, 20].

1.3. Comparison of autobioluminescent, traditional bioluminescent, and fluorescent optical imaging approaches

Unlike alternative bioluminescent and fluorescent reporter systems, which have been widely employed for drug discovery for many years, the autobioluminescent system is relatively new and thus has not been used by as many investigators as have the traditional systems. It is therefore important to briefly define the primary differences between these systems and detail the advantages and disadvantages of each as potential optical imaging targets. Fluorescent systems, with green fluorescent protein (*gfp*) being the most recognizable example, are arguably the most familiar of the optical imaging approaches and have several significant advantages in that they are small, single gene constructs that are simple to introduce into cells, do not require chemical exposure or sample destruction to function, and are available in a wide variety of excitation and emission wavelengths to suit individual assay needs [21]. Their primary drawback is that their requisite excitation signals can result in autofluorescent background signals from the cells or subjects under study, often requiring specialized equipment to filter out undesired light in order to acquire the resultant emission signal [22]. In addition, complications can arise from the prolongation of fluorescent protein activity after transcription has been stopped (enzymatically or through cell death) and phototoxicity to host cells, yielding inaccurate readings in toxicity or metabolic activity assays.

Bioluminescent reporters, on the other hand, express high signal-to-noise ratios due to the near absence of natural bioluminescent production from host tissues and can be sourced from a variety of different organisms with different substrates and output wavelengths to allow for reporter multiplexing within a single system. However, similar to fluorescent reporters, the luciferase proteins can remain active following genetic downregulation or cell death. In addition, the introduction of the activating chemical substrate has the potential to unexpectedly influence the cellular system under study and requires the destruction of the sample to efficiently interact with the genetically expressed luciferase [23].

Autobioluminescent reporters somewhat bridge these two systems by combining the favorable high signal-to-noise ratios of traditional bioluminescent systems and the nondestructive nature of the fluorescent systems. However, while their reliance on only endogenously produced substrates eliminates concerns over phototoxicity or substrate interference, it also reduces their total bioluminescent output levels relative to chemically stimulated systems. In addition, there is currently only a single variant, and thus only a single output signal wavelength, available for use [24]. Therefore, in the absence of a system that overcomes all limitations, investigators must weigh the pros and cons of each approach to determine which is the most appropriate for gathering their required data.

2. The use of autobioluminescent cellular models for high throughput compound screening

2.1. Advantages of autobioluminescent cellular models for high throughput screening

Despite their output limitations relative to chemically stimulated bioluminescent systems, autobioluminescent cellular models are particularly well suited for cytotoxicity assays and tier I drug development screening because of their ability to endogenously synthesize and regenerate the luminogenic substrates and cofactors ($FMNH_2$ and O_2) required for light production. This autonomous signal production potential eliminates costly reagents and minimizes the complexity of traditional assays formats, offering a simplified and cost-effective high throughput approach that reduces hands-on human interaction and error. In practice, the inherent high signal-to-noise ratio of the autobioluminescent signal is able to overcome the relatively reduced total output flux to allow these models to function similarly to their chemically stimulated counterparts [19, 25, 26]. This provides a significant advantage for their use in *in vitro* high throughput viability assays, which have traditionally been fluorescence based and are complicated by high background interference from cellular heme compounds and tissue culture supplements [26–29]. This reduction in background has allowed autobio-luminescent cellular models to be applied as counterscreens for identifying false positives in assays with notoriously high background effects, as was recently demonstrated in a study to assess the rate of false positives in a fluorescence-based assay for detecting the Alzheimer's-implicated Tau protein [30].

While this low background advantage is shared by traditional bioluminescent cellular models, the unstimulated production of light that is unique to the autobioluminescent system provides an additional advantage in that it allows for longitudinal data acquisition without sample destruction. The presence of a continuous output signal that can represent real-time metabolic activity dynamics offers enhanced temporal resolution for assaying the cytotoxicity of therapeutic compounds in high throughput screening formats and provides for standardiza-tion without the need to tailor each assay to the unknown kinetics of novel compounds [19].

The typical chemically stimulated, bioluminescent-based *in vitro* high throughput screening assay requires an average of five sacrificial time points to generate sufficient data for understanding the cytotoxicity of a compound. To take advantage of the full throughput capacity of a 1536-well plate, this requires the preparation, treatment, and processing of 7680 samples. However, the nondestructive nature of the autobioluminescent testing format reduces these sample requirements to only a single plate (1536 samples), which can then be imaged repeatedly at each time point. This eliminates the generation, maintenance, and treatment of 6144 samples over the course of a typical assay, and thus greatly reduces financial costs while increasing the convenience and quality of kinetic data collection.

2.2. Previously published examples of autobioluminescent cellular models for high throughput screening

Because of the reduction in cost and complexity and increase in data acquisition afforded by continuous imaging, autobioluminescent cellular models are becoming increasingly employed as tools for early stage therapeutic compound cytotoxicity screening. Recently, researchers at the National Institutes of Health performed a competitive evaluation of autobioluminescent and commonly applied ATP content, alamarBlue, CyQUANT, and MTS metabolic activity assays using a multi-time point study approach and reported that the IC_{50} data of known cytotoxic compounds were consistent across each system [25]. In this comparison, the continuous data output of the autobioluminescent cellular models was specifically investigated by comparing a single sample set against individually prepared sample sets that were sacrificed at each time point, and it was determined that repeated assessment of a single sample correlated well with the individually prepared samples of the alternative assays.

More in-depth comparisons have also been performed that contrasted the use of autobioluminescent and chemically stimulated bioluminescent reporter systems to assess the pharmacological effects of compounds on human cellular models *in vitro*. In this evaluation, the autobioluminescent models were compared with a chemically stimulated bioluminescent ATP content assay following exposure of cells to the Library of Pharmacologically Active Compounds (LOPAC), which contains 1280 compounds known to possess pharmacologically active effects on human tissues. When deployed in a high throughput 1536-well format, the IC_{50} data from the autobioluminescent cellular models yielded a strong correlation to the results of the ATP assay ($R^2 = 0.7847$), but with the added strength of allowing for kinetic monitoring, thus showcasing its power as a biomonitoring tool for cell toxicity and compatibility with high throughput conditions. While this study focused on the HEK293 human kidney cell line, the same advantages should remain applicable in more medically relevant drug screening models as well [19].

2.3. Incorporation of autobioluminescent cellular models into existing drug discovery workflows

Although it has not been the primary focus of any previously published autobioluminescent work, an interesting observation from the existing literature is that autobioluminescent cellular models can often be substituted into existing bioluminescent and fluorescent assay workflows without significant changes to the original assay protocols. This interoperability results from the similarity of the autobioluminescent output signal to those from the chemically simulated bioluminescent systems for which the protocols and existing detection equipment were originally designed. Because in both cases the output signals are light in the visible wavelength, the only major considerations when switching between systems have been the variation in output signal intensity and the necessary imaging parameter adjustments needed to achieve minimum signal detection thresholds. This minimizes the level of hardware optimization required to shift between assay modalities in both *in vitro* and *in vivo* imaging protocols.

A review of the literature suggests that the primary method for optimizing minimum signal detection thresholds during this transition has been to employ larger numbers of cells to overcome the difference in signal output between chemically stimulated and autobioluminescent systems. In autobioluminescent systems, signal detection has been demonstrated from population sizes down to 20,000 cells/well in a 24-well plate format, and from as few as 25,000 cells following subcutaneous injection into a mouse model [18]. While these are significantly larger numbers of cells than are required for chemically stimulated bioluminescent systems, the low background associated with bioluminescence has nonetheless been shown to retain sufficient sensitivity for use in whole-animal imaging experiments [28, 31]. It is important to note, however, that in some cases the use of increased cell numbers is not possible, such as for studies specifically focused on very small numbers of cells, such as early stage colonizing tumors. In these scenarios, the primary optimization employed must focus on adjustment of the imaging parameters, such as the use of longer acquisition times or increased luminescent pixel binning sizes.

3. Correlating the data output of autobioluminescent cellular models to classical assay formats

Since the generation of autobioluminescence relies upon the cell's capability to express the synthetic bacterial luciferase cassette as well as the availability of endogenous metabolites (e.g., O_2 and $FMNH_2$) for the synthesis of the required substrates, the autobioluminescent light output of these models correlates very strongly with the overall cellular metabolic activity level. As such, autobioluminescent cellular models represent excellent indicators for cytotoxicity following exposure to a compound of interest. Unlike conventional cytotoxicity assays that often require cellular destruction concurrent with data acquisition, autobioluminescent cellular models continuously self-modulate their light output in response to metabolic activity dynamics across the full lifetime of the host, thus allowing for the noninvasive visualization of metabolic activity at any time point throughout the entire exposure period. As a result, the nondestructive autobioluminescence assay generates more data similar to that obtained by traditional assays while simultaneously reducing the number of samples and investigator interaction time required per run. As an example of these capabilities, a side-by-side comparison between an autobioluminescent HEK293 cell model and the classic 3-(4,5-dimethylthiazol-2-yl)-2,5-diphenyltetrazolium bromide (MTT) cytotoxicity assay was performed over a 96-

hour exposure period. In this evaluation, the autobioluminescent model system demonstrated similar toxicity response data across the full set of compound exposure concentrations, and correlated strongly with the MTT assay (R^2 = 0.9262 at 96-hour postexposure) (**Figure 2A**). Similarly, a strong correlation (R^2 = 0.9163) was obtained between the autobioluminescent model system and an ATP content-based CellTiter-Glo cytotoxicity assay at 48-hour postexposure (**Figure 2B**). Although all these assays performed very similarly, it is important to note that the MTT and CellTiter-Glo assays both required individual sample sets to be prepared for each time point, whereas the substrate-free nature of the autobioluminescent cellular model system allowed for repeated monitoring of the same sample populations over time.

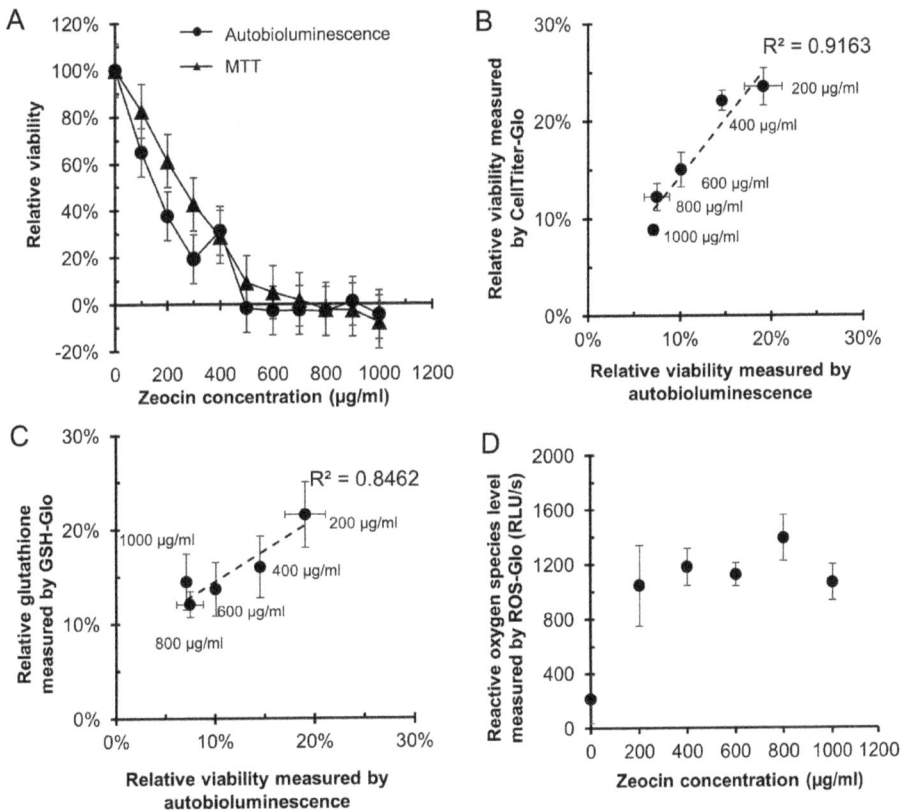

Figure 2. Correlating the data output of an autobioluminescent cellular model to alternative assay formats. (A) side-by-side comparison of the autobioluminescent model system output signal and the MTT cytotoxicity assay output for HEK293 cells exposed to 200–1000 μg/ml of Zeocin for 96 hours. (B) correlation of the relative viabilities of Zeocin-treated HEK293 cells as measured by autobioluminescence (x-axis) relative to those determined by the chemically stimulated bioluminescent CellTiter-Glo ATP content assay (y-axis). Each data point represents treatment with a unique dose of Zeocin. Relative viability was expressed as a percentage of the corresponding assay reading from untreated control cells. (C) correlation of the relative viabilities of Zeocin-treated HEK293 cells as measured by autobioluminescence (x-axis) relative to the chemically stimulated bioluminescent GSH-Glo glutathione concentration assay (y-axis). (D) treatment with 200–1000 μg/ml Zeocin resulted in an increase in reactive oxygen species levels in HEK293 cells that was not correlated to Zeocin concentration nor autobioluminescent output.

Furthermore, it was possible to leverage the nondestructive nature of the autobioluminescent HEK293 model to multiplex the real-time cytotoxicity assay with other downstream assays in order to further elucidate the specific toxicity pathways that were activated. To illustrate this application, following evaluation for metabolic activity by autobioluminescent output, the cells were then immediately assayed to measure intracellular glutathione levels using a GSH-Glo assay or for the presence of reactive oxygen species using a ROS-Glo assay. In these evaluations, the GSH-Glo and ROS-Glo assays, respectively, identified a reduction in gluta-thione concentration and an increase in reactive oxygen species level, indicating oxidative stress. However, only the reduction in glutathione concentration was determined to be dose responsive, and correlated with the reduction in autobioluminescent output with an R^2 value of 0.8462 across the full range of compound exposure concentrations (200–1000 µg/ml) (**Figure 2C**). In contrast, reactive oxygen species levels were not observed to correlate with either the test compound concentrations or the autobioluminescent output (**Figure 2D**).

4. Variability of autobioluminescent responses resulting from system expression in different cellular hosts

4.1. Demonstrated autobioluminescent cellular model systems

Thus far, only four autobioluminescent cellular models have been demonstrated: human kidney cells (HEK293) [10, 18], human liver cells (HepG2), immortalized breast cancer cells (T-47D) [19, 32], and colorectal cancer cells (HCT116) [19]. The most well documented of these models has been the HEK293 cell line, which underwent validation by the National Institutes of Health as a pharmaceutical screening tool [25]. Less documentation is available for the T-47D, HepG2, and HCT116 cell lines; however, an analysis of their previous use has indicated that their average autobioluminescent output levels are lower than that of their autobiolumi-nescent HEK293 counterpart [19], likely due to differences in their basal metabolic activity levels. Nonetheless, the signals from these alternative models have proven to be easily detectable [19], and their tumorigenic lineage has made them useful beyond the straightfor-ward toxicology/metabolic activity screening applications that have emerged as the primary role for the autobioluminescent HEK293 model.

In particular, the autobioluminescent T-47D model has found utility as a biomonitor for the detection of endocrine disruptor activity due to its natural proliferative rate increase following estrogenic compound exposure. Since estrogenic compounds are defined by their stimulation of cell reproduction, this model has been harnessed to assay for increases in autobiolumines-cent output as a function of cellular proliferation to track a compound's ability to function as an endocrine disruptor using automated imaging equipment [19, 32]. In this role, autobiolu-minescent T-47D cells were shown to exhibit output signals proportional to their total popu-lation size ($R^2 = 0.99$) across a large dynamic range, suggesting that this model is appropriate for estimating the changes in population size stimulated by estrogenic responses. When challenged with picomolar concentrations of the prototypical estrogenic chemical, 17β-estradiol, a dose-dependent autobioluminescent response similar to traditional cell prolifera-tion assays was observed [33]; however, contrary to the classical estrogenicity screens that require sample destruction, the autobioluminescent endocrine disruptor detection assay maintained its trademark benefit of continuous data collection without sample sacrifice. This made the platform an efficient and universal screening system that offered the continuous detection of both cell toxicity and estrogenicity without the additional reagent costs traditionally associated with assay multiplexing.

4.2. Variability of autobioluminescent responses across differential cellular models

Because the autobioluminescent phenotype is closely related to the metabolic activity level of the host cell expressing the synthetic bacterial luciferase cassette, it is possible that significant variances in signal output potential can exist among available cellular models. This concern is compounded by the nascent state of the technology, which has limited the number of cellular hosts documented in the literature and made it difficult to determine how consistent the reporter signal output strength will be upon expression in previously untested cell lines or tissues. The uncertainty surrounding this variability is concerning given that choosing an appropriate cellular model is particularly crucial in drug discovery applications where the same compound can exert variable toxicological responses in different cell lines or tissue types [34]. Due to the lack of published data on this topic, experiments were performed to compare the autobioluminescent responses of the HEK293, T-47D, and HepG2 cell lines following exposure to the common chemotherapeutic agent doxorubicin. Due to the nondestructive, continuous nature of these autobioluminescent cellular models, it was possible to track the impact of doxorubicin exposure on metabolic activity dynamics over a 72-hour exposure period. In this example, a typical sigmoidal dose response was observed from the HEK293 cells at each assay time point with an estimated IC_{50} value of 2×10^{-8} M (20 nM) at 72-hour postexposure (**Figure 3A**). However, doxorubicin treatment at concentrations higher than 5×10^{-7} M (500 nM) reduced autobioluminescent output by more than 95% within 72 hours of treatment. In contrast, both the T-47D and HepG2 models were less susceptible to doxorubicin than the HEK293 cells, and neither produced a sigmoidal dose response (**Figure 3B** and **C**). For these models, autobioluminescence reductions of greater than 95% were only observed by 72 hours following the start of doxorubicin treatment at concentrations ≥ 5 μM, whereas treatment with concentrations lower than 20 nM resulted in less than a 10% reduction in autobioluminescence output. Interestingly, however, doxorubicin treatment at 500 nM and 1 μM induced an increase

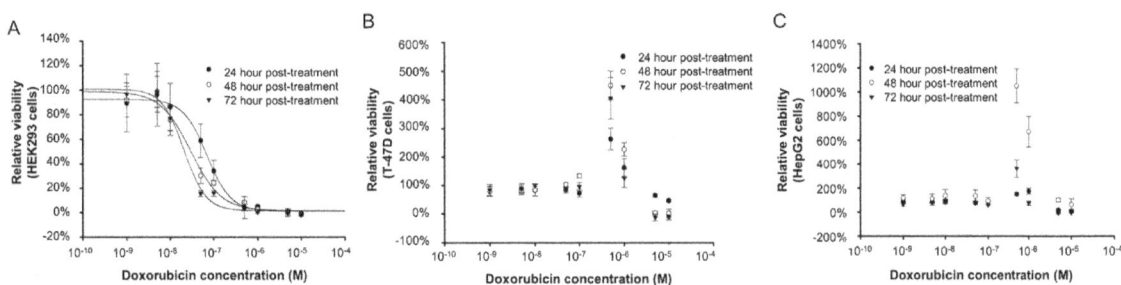

Figure 3. Variability of autobioluminescent dynamics in response to doxorubicin treatment across different cellular models. (A) autobioluminescent HEK293 cells displayed a sigmoidal dose-response curve in response to doxorubicin treatment at 24, 48, and 72 hours posttreatment. In contrast, neither (B) T-47D nor (C) HepG2 cells produced similar autobioluminescent responses to doxorubicin treatment over the course of the exposure period.

in autobioluminescent output in both the T-47D and HepG2 models over the course of the exposure period, with a peak at 48-hour posttreatment. These differential autobioluminescent responses are hypothesized to be the result of the varying cellular metabolic background activities and differential gene expression patterns exerted by each cell's activated toxicity pathways, thus demonstrating a clear emphasis on the importance of choosing a cellular model with an appropriate metabolic background for each specific application.

5. The use of autobioluminescent cellular models for three-dimensional cell culture applications

5.1. Common three-dimensional scaffold materials for *in vitro* drug discovery assays

Under natural *in vivo* conditions, cells reside in three-dimensional (3D) structures that are formed predominantly through attachment to an extracellular protein matrix. Partially through this attachment, the cells monitor and react to their immediate environment to modulate basic processes such as proliferation, morphology, and gene and protein expression, among other behaviors [35–37]. While in some cases, the natural proliferation rates and native phenotypes of the cells are retained under traditional monolayer culture conditions, more often their observed behavior and physiology become altered and are no longer representative of their natural *in vivo* characteristics [38]. In contrast, cells cultured in naturally derived or synthetically produced *in vitro* 3D culture systems have been demonstrated to better recapitulate *in vivo* cellular phenomena [39, 40]. Therefore, modern *in vitro* drug discovery platforms are increasingly taking advantage of synthetic 3D culture scaffolds to induce cellular growth under more *in vivo*-like conditions in order to improve the efficiency of novel compound development [41–43].

This transition has provided investigators with a variety of different 3D cell culture scaffold materials to choose from, many of which differ vastly in composition and, therefore, appropriateness to specific culture conditions. Collagen, a ubiquitous, naturally occurring protein polymer, has become frequently used for generalized *in vitro* 3D culture systems. The adaptability of collagen allows it to be used either on its own, as a hydrogel in which cells are suspended and then eventually attach to and remodel, or as a proteinaceous coating on other substrates [44]. Similar to collagen, other naturally occurring protein (e.g., fibrin or silks) and polysaccharide (e.g., chitin or hyaluronic acid) polymers have also been used alone, or in blends, to structure 3D cellular matrices [45] and affect cellular activities [46, 47]. In addition to these proteins, other natural materials such as corals have found utility as scaffolding for bone tissue engineering [48], as well as decellularized tissues repopulated with different cell types [49].

Synthetic polymers such as polycaprolactone, a comparatively basic example that is biodegradable and commonly used in medical applications, have also been widely applied toward 3D cell culture [50]. These synthetic 3D culture materials are becoming a popular option for *in vitro* drug discovery platforms due to their ability to be embedded with growth factors [51], specialized with functional groups, or studded with small molecules [52]. This generally offers investigators more options for tailoring the physical characteristics of the final scaffold, such as fiber traits, meshed patterns, sponge surface area, void volume, and more precise control of the final physical design.

5.2. The advantages of autobioluminescent systems for cellular screening in three-dimensional cell culture applications

Both fluorescent and bioluminescent imaging systems are easily employed for interrogating cellular structures and activities in traditional monolayer cultures, but the utility of both is handicapped within 3D cell culture systems [26, 53]. Fluorescent reporters are limited primarily by the materials used in 3D culture systems, most of which display high levels of autofluorescence as the scaffold material responds to the excitation signal, or in some cases, to the presence of ambient light [54]. This effect manifests as strong background noise that can completely eclipse the desired signal and is especially prevalent for collagen or collagen-coated scaffolds, which display autofluorescence around 420–460 nm [54]. Further compounding the use of fluorescent technologies in 3D culture are the effects of phototoxicity and photobleaching. The repeated bombardment of samples with excitation photon energy has been shown to increase the prevalence of reactive oxygen species, which in turn can damage cellular components and skew assay results to the point where the cells may no longer be representative of their true *in vivo* state [55, 56]. Photobleaching, on the other hand, occurs when the fluorescent reporter is destroyed by the input photon energy and is no longer available to release photons. This attenuates the output signal and diminishes assay sensitivity, resulting in potential data misinterpretation. In addition to these cellular concerns, the 3D cell culture scaffold itself can also interfere with excitation by presenting a physical barrier to photon excitation at the interior of a construct that can be tens to hundreds of micrometers thick. To compensate for this, investigators must apply increased excitation intensities or durations to reach acceptable signal-to-noise ratios, which in turn increase the prevalence of autofluorescence, phototoxicity, and photobleaching.

Because of these multiple hurdles to using fluorescent reporters in 3D culture systems, bioluminescence has become more prevalent as an imaging system under these conditions [54, 57]. However, traditional chemically stimulated bioluminescent systems are similarly limited by the tendency of the 3D scaffold material to induce heterogeneous substrate distribution. Unlike monolayer cultures, where the activating chemical can be evenly distributed to all cells in a population, the presence of the 3D scaffold material, and the variations in construct size, cell density, and matrix configuration across the scaffold, results in the uneven distribution of the activating chemical and its required cosubstrates [58]. Consequently, cells on the exterior of the scaffold have more efficient access to the activating chemical than those on the interior and therefore can initiate a luminescent signal with altered timing and kinetics. This can lead to ambiguous bioluminescent measurements across the population of cells under study and misrepresentations of the true state of the system [36].

Unlike these fluorescent and chemically stimulated bioluminescent systems, autobioluminescent cellular models produce their luminescent signals independent of any external stimulation, and therefore are not subject to limitations imposed by activating chemical diffusion dynamics, excitatory photon penetration, or phototoxicity and photobleaching. As a result, every cell in the population is continuously producing an autobioluminescent signal representative of its current metabolic activity level. Therefore, even if an asymmetric autobioluminescent signal is measured from a 3D construct, that distribution itself is of significant value to the investigator because it is an objective report on a cell's state at any given position in the construct. The primary physical limitation to the use of autobioluminescent cellular models within 3D culture conditions is the physical absorption and dispersion of the autobioluminescent signal as it interacts with the structural material. As with the alternative systems, this can be mediated through the selection of amenable scaffolding material or by increasing signal acquisition times in order to obtain increased photon counts, although it cannot be completely eliminated as it is a fundamental limitation of the use of 3D structures within the culture system itself.

5.3. Using autobioluminescent cellular models to elucidate metabolic activity and drug responsiveness in monolayer and three-dimensional culture systems

The choice between a traditional monolayer and a 3D cell culture platform can strongly influence the basal metabolic activity of the cells under study. In monolayer formats, the metabolic state of the cells is constantly in flux as they are continuously passaged until senescence. In contrast, cells seeded into a natural or synthetic 3D scaffold may proliferate initially but, over time, their growth rate will slow and they will enter a stabilized metabolic equilibrium [42, 59]. This growth format is more representative of the cells' natural state, as their proliferation rates, morphology, and gene expression more closely resemble their *in vivo* states [41–43, 60]. However, the use of a 3D culture system does not guarantee faithful replication of *in vivo*-like conditions, as the 3D scaffold itself, through traits such as matrix stiffness or construct dimensions, can induce hypoxia at levels that differ significantly from those observed *in vivo* [61, 62]. These cases often better model tumor biology than healthy tissues, with the 3D construct mimicking a necrotic center with a proliferative exterior and a range of metabolic states in between [63]. Therefore, the direct comparison of metabolic activity levels (whether under a steady state, during proliferation, or throughout viability transitions) between scaffold types, traditional monolayer cultures, and *in vivo* cells can be complicated and should be made while considering factors like nutrient gradients, surface area, cell density, and relative perfusion rates, among many others.

Given the contrasting metabolic conditions between monolayer and 3D cell culture systems, autobioluminescent cellular models are uniquely positioned to assess cellular health in ways other imaging modalities cannot. Since autobioluminescent cells produce light as a function of their individual metabolic state without a dependence on externally supplied activating chemicals or excitatory photon stimulation, cross-platform comparisons can be performed with limited uncontrollable variability and using sample preparation scales that are logistically tractable. Indeed, an investigation of these contrasts using autobioluminescent HEK293 cells seeded onto polycaprolactone 3D culture scaffolds demonstrated a higher proliferation rate and basal metabolic activity level than when an identical number of cells was seeded and grown in monolayers on polystyrene plates or in suspension culture [64]. Similarly, when a range of cellular concentrations were either plated in monolayers or encapsulated in collagen hydrogels and examined for autobioluminescence, only the output signals from the collagen-encapsulated 3D cultures remained tightly correlated with the initial cell density measurements after 48 hours of incubation. This suggests that, compared to traditional monolayer culture approaches, collagen-encapsulated 3D culture allows for longer term measurements of a wide range of cell population sizes.

Further interrogation indicated that the differences in basal metabolic levels induced by scaffold composition were significant enough to influence how the cells responded to xenobiotic challenges [42, 65], demonstrating that these emerging methods of 3D culture and adequate tools for evaluating cellular health are essential to modern drug discovery models. These results were not limited to only a single cell type, as breast, pancreatic and colon cancer cellular models all showed alterations to their proliferation and metabolic rates in the presence of stiffer 3D matrices, and were consequently found to be less sensitive to paclitaxel and gemcitabine treatment [62]. This was corroborated through a direct interrogation of collagen-encapsulated autobioluminescent HEK293 cells, which were observed to be more resistant to treatment with a metabolic inhibitor relative to their monolayer-grown counterparts. Together, these examples demonstrate how *in vitro* 3D culture alters cell behavior relative to traditional culture methods, and how investigators can use 3D culture variables to create better 3D models for drug discovery.

5.4. The use of autobioluminescent cellular models for continuous cellular tracking within three-dimensional culture scaffolds

Unlike fluorescent and chemically stimulated bioluminescent cellular models that require repeated, invasive stimulatory inputs to activate their output signals, autobioluminescent cellular models are amenable to continuous monitoring and dynamic metabolic activity tracking because their autobioluminescent output signals are continuously active. The on-demand availability and noninvasive nature of this output therefore makes these models highly amenable to repeated or continuous monitoring approaches that are not feasible with the traditional systems due to logistical or economical concerns. This offers significant utility for tumor xenograft tracking, which has traditionally relied upon repeated activating chemical injections, photonic stimulations, or physical measurements to track tumor volume, all of which are invasive and subject to large read-to-read variation [66, 67]. Autobioluminescent cellular models, in contrast, allow for low variation, high-resolution cellular tracking and viability monitoring.

As a demonstration of their utility for continuous monitoring, autobioluminescent HEK293 models have been grown on 3D polycaprolactone scaffolds and measured continuously for 24 hours via repeated light output measurements taken at 15-minute intervals using an automated system. Similarly, using magnetic-based 3D culture approaches, these same models have been monitored repeatedly for experiments lasting up to 45 days without the need to sacrifice samples or concerns related to sample-to-sample variability [64]. When employed in more complex *in vitro* 3D and xenograft models, the continuous signal generation of the autobioluminescent cellular models can be leveraged to provide data that was not previously obtainable, such as monitoring cell detachment from 3D constructs to model tumor metastasis. This approach has significant value for therapeutic and regenerative medicine applications, where tracking stem cells after implantation is currently difficult to implement, but critical for model development [68]. In this application, autobioluminescent stem cell models could be employed to continuously monitor the site of implantation for changes in cell number or health. Then, from within the same sample or animal subject, sloughed cells could be visualized at peripheral sites, such as the brain, because the cells remain autobioluminescent. This approach would offer significant advantages over chemically stimulated bioluminescent systems, whose activating chemicals cannot be evenly distributed to all tissues and are restricted from the brain by the blood-brain barrier.

6. Advantages of autobioluminescent cellular models for assaying the metabolic effects of nontraditional stressors

The autobioluminescent system's ability to initiate and self-modulate its signal generation without cellular destruction or exogenous substrate input gives it the ability to function fully intracellularly, which is significantly different than the majority of *in vitro* bioluminescent assays that employ the presence of intracellular metabolites, usually in the form of ATP, to act as a limiting reagent for supporting the bioluminescent production of an exogenously applied luciferase and excess required alternative cosubstrates. Functionally, this means that autobioluminescent systems can be utilized to monitor the metabolic activity or population size dynamics of specific community members in heterogeneous cocultures. This ability was recently investigated using cocultures of autobioluminescent HEK293 cells and virulent *Escherichia coli* O157:H7 to study the metabolic effects of bacterial infection and better understand the mechanism and timing of *E. coli* O157:H7 infection to improve treatment options for exposed patients [20].

In the course of this study, the autobioluminescent cellular system was compared to two other bioluminescence assays, the ATP-dependent CellTiter-Glo metabolic activity assay and the ROS-Glo hydrogen peroxide-dependent reactive oxygen species assay, in order to determine the most reliable method for assessing *E. coli* O157:H7 infection. Through the course of this evaluation, it was determined that the destructive assays were significantly influenced by the liberated metabolites from the co-lysed *E. coli* O157:H7 cells, which resulted in inflated readings due to overexposure of the exogenously supplemented luciferase reporter to the liberated bacterial metabolites. While the ATP-dependent CellTiter-Glo assay counterintuitively showed an increase in metabolic activity concurrent with cellular death, raising from 58.4% of uninfected control cell bioluminescence at 2-hour postinfection (hpi) to 70.8% by 4 hpi, the autobioluminescent system was self-limited to reporting only on the metabolic dynamics of the targeted human cellular population, which were shown to decrease from 11.2% of control cell autobioluminescence at 2 hpi to 2.5% by 4 hpi. Similar results were observed in comparisons between the autobioluminescent cellular model and the ROS-Glo assay, although no significant differences in reporter function were observed when uninfected control cells were compared across all three reporter systems [19, 25].

Using the autobioluminescent cellular model, the investigators were able to determine the minimum bacterial population threshold required to induce reductions in host cell metabolic activity to between 5×10^5 and 1×10^6 colony forming units. Additionally, the authors were able to leverage the nondestructive nature of the autobioluminescent cellular model to monitor the ability of the host cells to recover from *E. coli* O157:H7 infection by tracking metabolic activity continuously as the infecting bacteria were removed and antibacterial compounds were applied. This analysis allowed them to conclude that the host cells could return to normal metabolic activity within 2 hours of bacterial clearance, even after infections were allowed to reduce the basal metabolic activity of the cells to 2.6% of the untreated control cells. This study serves as a demonstrative example of the way that the autobioluminescent system can be applied to obtain data that would not be logistically or economically feasible to obtain using traditional chemically stimulated bioluminescent systems due to the large number of samples, significant hands-on time, and high reagent costs that would be required.

7. Expression of autobioluminescence using alternative host systems

Although not directly relevant to drug discovery, it is nonetheless important to note the significantly larger body of autobioluminescent work that has been performed in nonhuman model systems. Because the autobioluminescent gene cassette used for this work is the same as the one used for human cellular expression, only with alternative supporting genetic elements and codon optimization, it is highly likely that the techniques developed in these alternative models will eventually make their way into the autobioluminescent human cellular models as well. Based on historical development patterns, it is likely that the most impending modification to be constructed will be a chemically activated promoter system for compound-specific activation of autobioluminescent output. This approach has been used in both bacterial and yeast-based autobioluminescent models to assess transcriptional activity from reporter system-fused promoters [69], to monitor autobioluminescently tagged populations in the environment [70], and to detect environmental pollutants for bioremediation [71, 72].

The classical examples of this system are the *Saccharomyces cerevisiae*-based autobioluminescent estrogen (BLYES) [4] and androgen (BLYAS) [73] detection strains. These strains do not produce any signal in the absence of their activating signals, but can self-initiate luciferase expression in response to compound detection through the use of estrogen and androgen response elements, respectively. Their use of autobioluminescence as a reporter allows them to respond substantially faster than the traditional *lacZ*-based colorimetric screens, offering detectable autobioluminescence within 1–6 hours of exposure [73] compared to the 24-hour performance period of alternative *lacZ*-based reporter systems [74]. Although no drug discovery assays using this expression strategy have yet been reported in human cellular systems, the ability to initiate autobioluminescent production in response to promoter activation has been demonstrated, suggesting that these model formats are on the horizon [19].

8. Conclusions

Although autobioluminescent cellular models are a new technology, they have emerged as promising tools for drug discovery. Their ability to reduce the number of required sample preparation steps and reagent requirements for existing assay formats positions them well to lower assay costs, while their high signal-to-noise ratios can allow them to fill the nondestructive imaging gaps left by fluorescent systems with complicating levels of background autofluorescence. Similarly, their natural compatibility to work within complex 3D culture systems should, at least in the near term, make them robust against the upcoming shift toward this growth system for early stage compound evaluation. However, their ultimate utility as drug discovery tools will rely on their adoption by the investigators routinely performing these assays. Without widespread use, and therefore sufficient validation within the field, it will be difficult for these models to take hold regardless of the advantages they offer.

Acknowledgements

The authors acknowledge research funding provided by the U.S. National Institutes of Health under award numbers NIGMS-1R43GM112241-01A1, NIGMS-1R41GM116622-01, NIEHS-1R43ES026269-01, and NIEHS-2R44ES022567-02, the U.S. National Science Foundation under award number CBET-1530953, and the Oak Ridge National Laboratory Center for Nanophase Materials Sciences, which is a DOE Office of Science User Facility.

Author details

Tingting Xu[1], Michael Conway[2], Ashley Frank[2], Amelia Brumbaugh[2], Steven Ripp[1] and Dan Close[2*]

*Address all correspondence to: dan.close@490biotech.com

1 Center for Environmental Biotechnology, The University of Tennessee, Knoxville, USA

2 BioTech, Knoxville, Tennessee, USA

References

[1] Herring PJ. Systematic distribution of bioluminescence in living organisms. Journal of Bioluminescence and Chemiluminescence. 1987;1(3):147–163.

[2]   Close DM, Patterson SS, Ripp S, Baek SJ, Sanseverino J, Sayler GS. Autonomous bioluminescent expression of the bacterial luciferase gene cassette (*lux*) in a mammalian cell line. PLoS One. 2010;5(8):e12441.

[3]   King JMH, Digrazia PM, Applegate B, Burlage R, Sanseverino J, Dunbar P, et al. Rapid, sensitive bioluminescent reporter technology for naphthalene exposure and biodegradation. Science. 1990;249(4970):778–781.

[4]   Sanseverino J, Gupta RK, Layton AC, Patterson SS, Ripp SA, Saidak L, et al. Use of *Saccharomyces cerevisiae* BLYES expressing bacterial bioluminescence for rapid, sensitive detection of estrogenic compounds. Applied and Environmental Microbiology. 2005;71(8):4455–4460.

[5]   Coutant EP, Janin YL. Synthetic routes to coelenterazine and other imidazo [1, 2-a] pyrazin-3-one luciferins: Essential tools for bioluminescence-based investigations. Chemistry—A European Journal. 2015;21(48):17158–17171.

[6]   Close DM, Ripp S, Sayler GS. Reporter proteins in whole-cell optical bioreporter detection systems, biosensor integrations, and biosensing applications. Sensors. 2009;9(11):9147–9174.

[7]   Close D, Ripp S, Sayler GS. Mammalian-based bioreporter targets: Protein expression for bioluminescent and fluorescent detection in the mammalian cellular background. In: Serra P, editor. Biosensors for Health, Environment and Biosecurity. Rijeka, Croatia: Intech; 2011. pp. 469–498.

[8]   Sambrook J, Russell DW. Molecular Cloning: A Laboratory Manual. Cold Spring Harbor, New York: Cold Spring Harbor Laboratory Press; 2001.

[9]   Gould SJ, Subramani S. Firefly luciferase as a tool in molecular and cell biology. Analytical Biochemistry. 1988;175(1):5–13.

[10] Patterson SS, Dionisi HM, Gupta RK, Sayler GS. Codon optimization of bacterial luciferase (*lux*) for expression in mammalian cells. Journal of Industrial Microbiology & Biotechnology. 2005;32:115–123.

[11] Almashanu S, Musafia B, Hadar R, Suissa M, Kuhn J. Fusion of *luxA* and *luxB* and its expression in *E. coli*, *S. cerevisiae* and *D. melanogaster*. Journal of Bioluminescence and Chemiluminescence. 1990;5(2):89–97.

[12] Escher A, O'Kane DJ, Lee J, Szalay AA. Bacterial luciferase alpha beta fusion protein is fully active as a monomer and highly sensitive *in vivo* to elevated temperature. Proceedings of the National Academy of Sciences of the United States of America. 1989;86(17):6528–6532.

[13] Kirchner G, Roberts JL, Gustafson GD, Ingolia TD. Active bacterial luciferase from a fused gene: Expression of a *Vibrio harveyi luxAB* translational fusion in bacteria, yeast and plant cells. Gene. 1989;81(2):349–354.

[14] Koncz C, Olsson O, Langridge WH, Schell J, Szalay AA. Expression and assembly of functional bacterial luciferase in plants. Proceedings of the National Academy of Sciences of the United States of America. 1987;84(1):131–135.

[15] Olsson O, Escher A, Sandberg G, Schell J, Koncz C, Szalay AA. Engineering of monomeric bacterial luciferase by fusion of *luxA* and *luxB* genes in *Vibrio harveyi*. Gene. 1989;81(2):335–347.

[16] Pazzagli M, Devine JH, Peterson DO, Baldwin TO. Use of bacterial and firefly luciferases as reporter genes in DEAE-dextran-mediated transfection in mammalian cells. Analytical Biochemistry. 1992;204(2):315–323.

[17] Westerlund-Karlsson A, Saviranta P, Karp M. Generation of thermostable monomeric luciferases from *Photorhabdus luminescens*. Biochemical and Biophysical Research Communications. 2002;296(5):1072–1076.

[18] Close DM, Patterson SS, Ripp SA, Baek SJ, Sanseverino J, Sayler GS. Autonomous bioluminescent expression of the bacterial luciferase gene cassette (*lux*) in a mammalian cell line. PLoS One. 2010;5(8):e12441.

[19] Xu T, Ripp SA, Sayler GS, Close DM. Expression of a humanized viral 2A-mediated *lux* operon efficiently generates autonomous bioluminescence in human cells. PLoS One. 2014;9(5):e96347.

[20] Xu T, Marr E, Lam H, Ripp S, Sayler G, Close D. Real-time toxicity and metabolic activity tracking of human cells exposed to *Escherichia coli* O157:H7 in a mixed consortia. Ecotoxicology. 2015;24(10):2133–2140.

[21] Shaner NC, Steinbach PA, Tsien RY. A guide to choosing fluorescent proteins. Nature Methods. 2005;2(12):905–909.

[22] Close DM, Ripp SA, Sayler GS. Reporter proteins in whole-cell optical bioreporter detection systems, biosensor integrations, and biosensing applications. Sensors. 2009;9(11):9147–9174.

[23] Thorne N, Inglese J, Auld DS. Illuminating insights into firefly luciferase and other bioluminescent reporters used in chemical biology. Chemistry & Biology. 2010;17(6): 646–657.

[24] Xu T, Close D, Handagama W, Marr E, Sayler G, Ripp S. The expanding toolbox of *in vivo* bioluminescent imaging. Frontiers in Oncology. 2016;6:150.

[25] Class B, Thorne N, Aguisanda F, Southall N, Mckew J, Zheng W. High-throughput viability assay using an autonomously bioluminescent cell line with a bacterial *lux* reporter. Journal of Laboratory Automation. 2015;20(2):164–174.

[26] Close DM, Hahn RE, Patterson SS, Ripp SA, Sayler GS. Comparison of human optimized bacterial luciferase, firefly luciferase, and green fluorescent protein for contin-

uous imaging of cell culture and animal models. Journal of Biomedical Optics. 2011;16(4):e12441.

[27] Choy G, O'Connor S, Diehn FE, Costouros N, Alexaner HR, Choyke P, et al. Comparison of noninvasive fluorescent and bioluminescent small animal optical imaging. Biotechniques. 2003;35(5):1022–1030.

[28] Troy T, Jekic-McMullen D, Sambucetti L, Rice B. Quantitative comparison of the sensitivity of detection of fluorescent and bioluminescent reporters in animal models. Molecular Imaging. 2004;3(1):9–23.

[29] Welsh DK, Kay SA. Bioluminescence imaging in living organisms. Current Opinion in Biotechnology. 2005;16(1):73–78.

[30] Dehdashti SJ, Zheng W, Gever JR, Wilhelm R, Nguyen DT, Sittampalam G, et al. A high-throughput screening assay for determining cellular levels of total tau protein. Current Alzheimer Research. 2013;10(7):679–687.

[31] Zhao H, Doyle TC, Coquoz O, Kalish F, Rice BW, Contag CH. Emission spectra of bioluminescent reporters and interaction with mammalian tissue determine the sensitivity of detection *in vivo*. Journal of Biomedical Optics. 2005;10(4):41210.

[32] Xu T, Close DM, Webb JD, Price SL, Ripp SA, Sayler GS. Continuous, real-time bioimaging of chemical bioavailability and toxicology using autonomously bioluminescent human cell lines. In: SPIE-Sensing Technologies for Global Health, Military Medicine, Disaster Response and Environmental Monitoring III; 29 April–3 May, 2013. Baltimore, Maryland, USA. Berlingham, Washington: SPIE; 2013. p. 872310.

[33] Soto AM, Maffini MV, Schaeberle CM, Sonnenschein C. Strengths and weaknesses of *in vitro* assays for estrogenic and androgenic activity. Best Practice & Research Clinical Endocrinology & Metabolism. 2006;20(1):15–33.

[34] Holliday DL, Speirs V. Choosing the right cell line for breast cancer research. Breast Cancer Research. 2011;13(4):215–215.

[35] Khalil AA, Jameson MJ, Broaddus WC, Lin PS, Dever SM, Golding SE, et al. The influence of hypoxia and pH on bioluminescence imaging of luciferase-transfected tumor cells and xenografts. International Journal of Molecular Imaging. 2013;2013:9.

[36] Lambrechts D, Roeffaers M, Goossens K, Hofkens J, Vande Velde G, Van de Putte T, et al. A causal relation between bioluminescence and oxygen to quantify the cell niche. PLoS One. 2014;9(5):e97572.

[37] Kleinman HK, Philp D, Hoffman MP. Role of the extracellular matrix in morphogenesis. Current Opinion in Biotechnology. 2003;14(5):526–532.

[38] Pampaloni F, Reynaud EG, Stelzer EH. The third dimension bridges the gap between cell culture and live tissue. Nature Reviews Molecular Cell Biology. 2007;8(10):839–845.

[39] Berthiaume F, Moghe PV, Toner M, Yarmush ML. Effect of extracellular matrix topology on cell structure, function, and physiological responsiveness: Hepatocytes cultured in a sandwich configuration. The FASEB Journal. 1996;10(13):1471–1484.

[40] Cukierman E, Pankov R, Stevens DR, Yamada KM. Taking cell-matrix adhesions to the third dimension. Science. 2001;294(5547):1708–1712.

[41] Nam KH, Smith AS, Lone S, Kwon S, Kim DH. Biomimetic 3D tissue models for advanced high-throughput drug screening. Journal of Laboratory Automation. 2015;20(3):201–215.

[42] Edmondson R, Broglie JJ, Adcock AF, Yang L. Three-dimensional cell culture systems and their applications in drug discovery and cell-based biosensors. Assay and Drug Development Technologies. 2014;12(4):207–218.

[43] Breslin S, O'Driscoll L. Three-dimensional cell culture: The missing link in drug discovery. Drug Discovery Today. 2013;18(5–6):240–249.

[44] Chevallay B, Herbage D. Collagen-based biomaterials as 3D scaffold for cell cultures: Applications for tissue engineering and gene therapy. Medical & Biological Engineering & Computing. 2000;38(2):211–218.

[45] Taylor PM. Biological matrices and bionanotechnology. Philosophical Transactions of the Royal Society of London B: Biological Sciences. 2007;362(1484):1313–1320.

[46] Ruedinger F, Lavrentieva A, Blume C, Pepelanova I, Scheper T. Hydrogels for 3D mammalian cell culture: A starting guide for laboratory practice. Applied Microbiology and Biotechnology. 2015;99(2):623–636.

[47] Caliari SR, Burdick JA. A practical guide to hydrogels for cell culture. Nature Methods. 2016;13(5):405–414.

[48] Hou R, Chen F, Yang Y, Cheng X, Gao Z, Yang HO, et al. Comparative study between coral-mesenchymal stem cells-rhBMP-2 composite and auto-bone-graft in rabbit critical-sized cranial defect model. Journal of Biomedical Materials Research Part A. 2007;80(1):85–93.

[49] Hoshiba T, Lu H, Kawazoe N, Chen G. Decellularized matrices for tissue engineering. Expert Opinion on Biological Therapy. 2010;10(12):1717–1728.

[50] Dash TK, Konkimalla VB. Poly-ϵ-caprolactone based formulations for drug delivery and tissue engineering: A review. Journal of Controlled Release. 2012;158(1):15–33.

[51] Cetinkaya G, Turkoglu H, Arat S, Odaman H, Onur MA, Gumusderelioglu M, et al. LIF-immobilized nonwoven polyester fabrics for cultivation of murine embryonic stem cells. Journal of Biomedical Materials Research Part A. 2007;81(4):911–919.

[52] Vasita R, Katti DS. Nanofibers and their applications in tissue engineering. International Journal of Nanomedicine. 2006;1(1):15–30.

[53] White NS, Errington RJ. Fluorescence techniques for drug delivery research: Theory and practice. Advanced Drug Delivery Reviews. 2005;57(1):17–42.

[54] Smith LE, Smallwood R, Macneil S. A comparison of imaging methodologies for 3D tissue engineering. Microscopy Research and Technique. 2010;73(12):1123–1133.

[55] Daddysman MK, Tycon MA, Fecko CJ. Photoinduced damage resulting from fluorescence imaging of live cells. Methods in Molecular Biology. 2014;1148:1–17.

[56] Magidson V, Khodjakov A. Circumventing photodamage in live-cell microscopy. Methods in Cell Biology. 2013;114:545–560.

[57] Michelini E, Cevenini L, Calabretta MM, Calabria D, Roda A. Exploiting *in vitro* and *in vivo* bioluminescence for the implementation of the three Rs principle (replacement, reduction and refinement) in drug discovery. Analytical and Bioanalytical Chemistry. 2014;406(23):5531–5539.

[58] Malda J, Klein TJ, Upton Z. The roles of hypoxia in the *in vitro* engineering of tissues. Tissue Engineering. 2007;13(9):2153–2162.

[59] Wrzesinski K, Rogowska-Wrzesinska A, Kanlaya R, Borkowski K, Schwammle V, Dai J, et al. The cultural divide: Exponential growth in classical 2D and metabolic equilibrium in 3D environments. PLoS One. 2014;9(9):e106973.

[60] Birgersdotter A, Sandberg R, Ernberg I. Gene expression perturbation *in vitro*—A growing case for three-dimensional (3D) culture systems. Seminars in Cancer Biology. 2005;15(5):405–412.

[61] Pruksakorn D, Lirdprapamongkol K, Chokchaichamnankit D, Subhasitanont P, Chiablaem K, Svasti J, et al. Metabolic alteration of HepG2 in scaffold-based 3-D culture: Proteomic approach. Proteomics. 2010;10(21):3896–3904.

[62] Fang JY, Tan SJ, Wu YC, Yang Z, Hoang BX, Han B. From competency to dormancy: A 3D model to study cancer cells and drug responsiveness. Journal of Translational Medicine. 2016;14:38.

[63] Mehta G, Hsiao AY, Ingram M, Luker GD, Takayama S. Opportunities and challenges for use of tumor spheroids as models to test drug delivery and efficacy. Journal of Controlled Release. 2012;164(2):192–204.

[64] Webb JD. Evaluation of novel multi-dimensional tissue culturing methods using autonomously bioluminescent human cell lines [thesis]. Knoxville: The University of Tennessee; 2014.

[65] LaBonia GJ, Lockwood SY, Heller AA, Spence DM, Hummon AB. Drug penetration and metabolism in 3D cell cultures treated in a 3D printed fluidic device: Assessment of irinotecan via MALDI imaging mass spectrometry. Proteomics. 2016;16(11–12):1814–1821.

[66] Tomayko MM, Reynolds CP. Determination of subcutaneous tumor size in athymic (nude) mice. Cancer Chemotherapy and Pharmacology. 1989;24(3):148–154.

[67] Jenkins DE, Oei Y, Hornig YS, Yu SF, Dusich J, Purchio T, et al. Bioluminescent imaging (BLI) to improve and refine traditional murine models of tumor growth and metastasis. Clinical and Experimental Metastasis. 2003;20(8):733–744.

[68] von der Haar K, Lavrentieva A, Stahl F, Scheper T, Blume C. Lost signature: Progress and failures in *in vivo* tracking of implanted stem cells. Applied Microbiology and Biotechnology. 2015;99(23):9907–9922.

[69] Engebrecht J, Simon M, Silverman M. Measuring gene expression with light. Science. 1985;227(4692):1345–1347.

[70] de Weger LA, Dunbar P, Mahafee WF, Lugtenberg BJJ, Sayler GS. Use of bioluminescence markers to detect *Pseudomonas* spp. in the rhizosphere. Applied and Environmental Microbiology. 1991;57(12):3641–3644.

[71] Ripp S, Nivens DE, Ahn Y, Werner C, Jarrell J, Easter JP, et al. Controlled field release of a bioluminescent genetically engineered microorganism for bioremediation process monitoring and control. Environmental Science & Technology. 2000;34(5):846–853.

[72] Xu T, Close D, Smartt A, Ripp S, Sayler G. Detection of organic compounds with whole-cell bioluminescent bioassays. In: Thouand G, Marks R, editors. Bioluminescence: Fundamentals and Applications in Biotechnology, Volume 1. Advances in Biochemical Engineering/Biotechnology. 144. Berlin, Heidelberg: Springer; 2014. pp. 111–151.

[73] Eldridge M, Sanseverino J, Layton A, Easter J, Schultz T, Sayler G. *Saccharomyces cerevisiae* BLYAS, a new bioluminescent bioreporter for detection of androgenic compounds. Applied and Environmental Microbiology. 2007;73(19):6012–6018.

[74] Gaido KW, Leonard LS, Lovell S, Gould JC, Babai D, Portier CJ, et al. Evaluation of chemicals with endocrine modulating activity in a yeast-based steroid hormone receptor gene transcription assay. Toxicology and Applied Pharmacology. 1997;143(1): 205–212.

4

Job and Career Opportunities in the Pharmaceutical Sector

Josse R. Thomas, Chris van Schravendijk,

Lucia Smit and Luciano Saso

Additional information is available at the end of the chapter

Abstract

The pharmaceutical field offers a wealth of job and career opportunities for talented young graduates with a sound background in life sciences and various other academic disciplines. Because these employment options are often insufficiently known to young academics, the aim of this chapter is to give them a better idea about the many job opportunities and presents the entire drug life cycle. The first part of the chapter includes a general description of the drug life cycle and what is understood by 'the pharmaceutical sector'. The core of the chapter gives an overview of job opportunities that either are specific to the different parts of the drug life cycle or are important as support functions over the entire life cycle. It also includes a section on career perspectives and training opportunities. The last part of the chapter focuses on important employability elements, as well as some practical do's and don'ts for effective job application.

Keywords: job, career, drug discovery and development, pharmaceutical sector

1. Introduction

The field of drug discovery, development and commercialisation offers a wealth of job and career opportunities for talented young graduates with a sound background in life sciences or other academic disciplines and a genuine interest and motivation to start a professional career in the pharmaceutical sector.

The drug life cycle is usually subdivided into discovery research, development and commercialisation and spans the whole trajectory from idea to patients, from bench to market (withdrawal).

The professional field covers the whole pharmaceutical sector, which is not just limited to drugs or to medicines for human or animal use but also includes medical devices, diagnostics, radiopharmaceuticals, nutriceuticals and other related areas of activity. Nor is this sector limited to the (bio-)pharmaceutical industry, but it also includes health authorities, academia and research centres, clinical investigator sites, contract research organisations (CROs) and many more. The need for a highly educated workforce is clearly present in all of these areas and the pharma sector is offering opportunities for a wide spectrum of academic graduates with a Bachelor, a Master, or a PhD degree. Despite the many job opportunities in this sector, competencies of young university graduates are seldom adjusted to the specific requirements listed in the job vacancies. Moreover, they often lack an understanding of the drug development process and the various perspectives it offers for career development.

The aim of this chapter is to give academic graduates a better idea about the many job opportunities over the entire drug life cycle, offered by a wide variety of companies and organisations and for a broad spectrum of qualified professionals.

All the above will be presented in more detail in Sections 2–5 of this chapter.

After the overview of job opportunities, career perspectives and training opportunities will be discussed in Sections 6 and 7 and important employability elements in Section 8.

As this chapter is primarily targeted at young graduates, Section 9 adds some practical dos and don'ts for effective job application. The chapter ends with some concluding remarks (Section 10) and a bibliography for further reading.

2. The drug life cycle

The life cycle of a drug involves essentially three parts: drug discovery and design (research), drug development and drug commercialisation [1]. They are largely consecutive in nature, but some activities are carried out in parallel.

Drug research is primarily driven by an unmet medical need, i.e. a therapeutic area in need of a (better) drug. Drugs are either discovered in nature or in existing chemical libraries, or either (semi-)synthesised or designed *de novo* in laboratories. Drug discovery research and drug design require highly intellectual creativity, perseverance and some serendipity. As drugs interact with molecular targets of biological relevance for a disease, mostly proteins (such as receptors, enzymes, ion channels, or antigens), drug research requires intense collaboration between project team members of several scientific disciplines (such as biologists, medicinal chemists and pharmacologists). Drug discovery and design are characterised by a fairly high degree of freedom. It is mostly done in (big) pharmaceutical companies, academic research centres, as well as in small spin-offs and start-ups. The ultimate goal of the research project team is to deliver a (few) patented drug candidate(s), ready for development. This can take 3–5 years.

During drug development, the potential drug candidate progresses to a drug or a medicinal product which is effective and safe to be administered to humans (or animals) to prevent, diagnose, or treat a disease. It is a complex and highly regulated process, with a lot of intermediate failures, (re-)assessments and (re-)iterations along the long road. Because of these characteristics, drug development is often subdivided in non-clinical and clinical development, as well as in early and late development. In drug development for humans, clinical development includes all experiments with the drug in human subjects (healthy volunteers or patients), while non-clinical development includes all experiments with the drug in animals, *in vitro* and *in silico*. Non-clinical development consists of chemical and pharmaceutical development (of the drug product as a formulation, such as a tablet or an injectable solution), non-clinical efficacy and safety pharmacology, non-clinical toxicology and non-clinical pharmacokinetics. Non-clinical development is partly preclinical, i.e. some of it has to be performed and has to generate safe results before (a certain phase in) clinical development can start. Clinical development is classically divided into consecutive phases: phase 1 (first administration in man, single and multiple ascending dose studies, mostly in healthy volunteers), phase 2 (proof of concept that the drug has the intended effect in patients with the targeted disease, dose-finding studies), phase 3 (confirmation of efficacy and safety in clinical trials with large groups of patients), phase 4 (real-world studies when the drug is on the market, pharmacovigilance). Alternatively, clinical development is also split into an exploratory and a confirmatory phase, or a preapproval (before market authorisation) and a post-approval phase. Drug development is a highly risky and costly process; it takes easily 5–8 years and a very talented team of several disciplines (different life scientists, clinicians, engineers, regulatory affairs experts and others), all working together to make it a successful enterprise.

The final part, drug commercialisation, starts with the market authorisation (or drug approval), based on all the available data about quality, efficacy and safety on the medicine and a positive benefit-risk balance in the targeted population, allowing the drug to be marketed and to generate return on investment. But market authorisation (per country, per region like the European Union, or worldwide) is not enough to be successful on the market; there are other hurdles to be taken such as a fair price setting and drug reimbursement by social security systems (based on the added value of the drug for patients and its affordability by society), together known as market access hurdles. Once taken, the drug can be launched and marketing and sales can really start, in parallel with large-scale production and distribution. When the patent of the drug expires (generally 20 years after its application), generic and biosimilar competitors enter the market and the sales of the original drug suddenly drop (the patent cliff), but a drug with added value can still stay on the market for many more years, until it is finally withdrawn. Drug commercialisation is more a world of health economists, marketers, pharmacists, pharmaceutical physicians, sales reps, lawyers and business managers. A schematic representation of the drug life cycle is given in **Figure 1**.

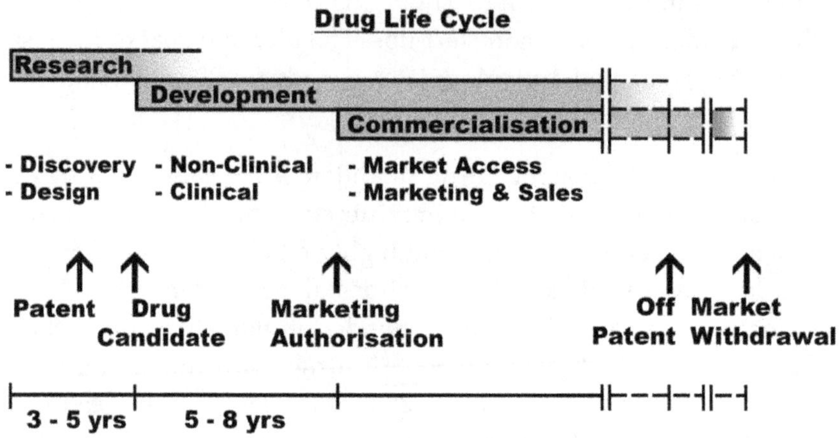

Drug Life Cycle

Figure 1. Schematic representation of the drug life cycle. yrs, years.

3. The pharmaceutical sector

The (bio-)pharmaceutical industry is probably the biggest employer in this sector worldwide.

It is already a world in itself, as it is an umbrella term with its main representatives being 'big pharma' companies, active throughout the whole value chain of the drug life cycle. They research, develop, manufacture and market innovative medicines, either the more classic small molecules or the more recently introduced large biopharmaceuticals such as therapeutic proteins and monoclonal antibodies (produced by living organisms or cells). Under the umbrella also operate medtech companies (e.g. medical devices, implants, biomaterials and *in vitro* diagnostics); biotech companies specialised in biopharmaceuticals, but also in advanced therapy medicinal products (ATMPs) such as gene and cell therapy, or tissue-engineered products; small- and medium-sized enterprises (SMEs) often as niche players; start- or scale-up companies more focused on drug research and early development; companies producing generics and biosimilars; organizations representing the pharmaceutical industry, such as *Ph*RMA in the USA and EFPIA in Europe; and last but not least, the ever growing business of Contract Research Organizations (CROs) as full or specific service providers to this industry.

However, the pharmaceutical sector is a lot broader than the pharmaceutical industry and offers many additional jobs and career opportunities. Other important organisations, institutions, or actors in this sector are regulatory agencies, such as national or regional medicines agencies (such as the FDA in the USA and the EMA in Europe, granting drug approvals), certified bodies (the equivalent for medical devices), or patent offices; academia, research centres and spin-offs active in basic research, drug discovery and design, but also early drug development; clinical investigator sites, be it phase 1 or clinical pharmacology units (CPUs) either university- or CRO-owned, university or regional hospitals, site management organisations (SMOs), or the European Organisation for the Research and Treatment of Cancer (EORTC); patient organisations; non-profit drug research funders such as the Bill and Melinda Gates Foundation; consultants, lobbyists and law firms; venture capitalists and investment banks; entrepreneurs and self-employed persons; and many more…

Overall, the pharmaceutical sector offers a wealth of job opportunities and career perspectives for young and talented graduates of the necessary calibre and commitment.

4. Job opportunities throughout the drug life cycle

In this section, we walk through the drug life cycle and focus on job opportunities that are specific to the different parts of the cycle. Support functions that are important over the entire cycle are presented in Section 5.

4.1. Discovery research

Drug discovery research is either phenotypic-based (empirical and response-driven) or target-based (molecular and hypothesis-driven). Although the phenotypic-based approach has been very successful in the past, today's drug discovery is more target-based. The process is as follows: (1) selection and validation of a (druggable) target, mostly a protein (e.g. receptor, enzyme, ion-channel and antigen), but also carriers of genetic information (e.g. DNA/RNA and oncogenes); (2) development and validation of a proper assay, allowing to study the interaction between the target and potential drug candidates; (3) (high-throughput) screening (HTS) of potential drugs, generated through *de novo* synthesis or from existing natural or chemical libraries, in order to identify 'hits' (interactions with the target); (4) hit-to-lead finding, i.e. limited optimisation of drug candidates in order to identify a limited number of promising lead compounds; (5) lead optimisation, with the objective to improve target selectivity and specificity, as well as the pharmacodynamic, pharmacokinetic and toxicological properties of the candidate drug, in order to get it ready for development.

Drug discovery research is highly dependent on the interplay between different scientific and other disciplines. In practice, it includes intensive collaboration between mainly:

- different types of biologists, such as molecular biologists, biochemists, biotechnologists, bioinformaticians and biomedical scientists;

- different types of chemists, such as medicinal chemists, combichem specialists, computer-assisted drug designers, protein chemists and analytical chemists;

- pharmacologists, pharmacokineticists, pharmacometricians, toxicologists, biopharmacy and pharmaceutical technology experts;

- as well as representatives of other disciplines, such as (bio-)engineers, data analysts, intellectual property (IP) specialists and patent lawyers.

Drug research departments may be organised per therapeutic domain (more specialised and more compartmentalised) or rather more 'holistically' per biological platform, such as a similar target family (e.g. kinases and ion channels), or a similar biological mechanism (e.g. angiogenesis, inflammation, cell cycle control and epigenetics), or per common technological platform (e.g. 3D modelling, X-ray crystallography and NMR spectroscopy).

Innovative drug research organisations (pharmaceutical companies, academic centres, spin-offs, or start-ups) are looking for highly educated and talented individuals with at least a master's degree and preferably a PhD in the aforementioned disciplines. However, being an excellent scientist is not enough to be successful in this field. You also need the right creative mindset, being able to think out of the box and to work together in a multidisciplinary team on a specific project for several years.

Discovery research is the least regulated phase of the drug life cycle and confers to professionals working in this field a fairly high degree of freedom, although in the competitive world of today, research teams also have to deliver quality products, in time and within budget.

As drug R&D is costly and risky; drug candidates are patented so that they later gain market exclusivity without competition for a set period (in general, 20 years after patent filing). Therefore, drug research organisations as well as national and international patent offices also offer job opportunities for IP specialists, such as patent lawyers and patent reviewers.

4.2. Non-clinical development

Non-clinical drug development, including all experiments not involving human subjects, is an umbrella term referring to the following activities: chemical and pharmaceutical development (also known as 'chempharm' or 'chemistry, manufacturing and controls (CMC)'), experimental pharmacology (including safety pharmacology), non-clinical toxicology and non-clinical pharmacokinetics. It is essentially a lab activity, involving *in vitro* and *in silico* research as well as animal experiments. Its goal is to generate the data needed as prerequisites for the different clinical development phases (the preclinical part of non-clinical development), all the non-clinical data for the marketing authorisation application (the preapproval phase), as well as all the non-clinical data during the continued development when the drug is already on the market (the post-approval phase). Non-clinical development is much more regulated than discovery research and has to be executed within a framework of international guidelines (ICH Quality and Safety guidelines) and according to the international standards of good laboratory or good manufacturing practices (GLP and GMP).

Chemical and pharmaceutical development, including drug (product) manufacturing and drug (product) analysis, offers opportunities especially for analytical and green chemists, chemical or bio-engineers, pharmaceutical technologists and (industrial) pharmacists.

Non-clinical efficacy and safety pharmacology units are rather looking for experimental pharmacologists, biomedical, or (bio-)pharmaceutical scientists.

Non-clinical pharmaceutical toxicology departments are essentially in need of toxicologists, veterinary surgeons and pathologists, but can also do well with interested biomedical or (bio-)pharmaceutical scientists.

Non-clinical pharmacokinetics departments are especially looking for pharmacokineticists, experts in drug metabolism and bio-analytical chemists. As model-based drug development is booming, there is also a high need for pharmacometricians, modelling and simulation experts, or more generally, biomedical or (bio-)pharmaceutical scientists with a sound background in mathematics.

For most executive functions in all the above-cited fields, having a master's degree is an absolute must and a PhD a big plus, although a lot of lab technicians are also welcome.

Non-clinical drug development specialists are also needed in (inter-)national medicines agencies as assessors of the CMC (quality) and the non-clinical (safety) parts of the common technical document (CTD), the international harmonised dossier for application of a marketing authorisation of pharmaceuticals for human and animal use.

4.3. Clinical development

Clinical drug development, defined as all studies involving human subjects, is (because of its complexity and long duration) usually subdivided into different phases. It starts classically with small-scale phase 1 studies, including the First-in-Man or First-in-Human (FiM/FiH) study, the single ascending dose (SAD) and the multiple ascending dose (MAD) studies, usually in healthy volunteers (but sometimes in patients), in order to have a first impression of the safety, pharmacokinetics and pharmacodynamics of the drug in development in humans. Then follows phase 2a, to investigate whether the drug works at all in patients according to the presumed mechanism of action (the so-called Proof-of-Concept or POC study) and to have a preliminary idea about the effective and safe dose range in tens of patients with the intended indication. Nowadays, phase 1 is often preceded by a phase 0 study with a limited number of subjects, with a single radioactive microdose of a limited number of drug candidates in order to help researchers in the selection of the best candidate for further full development. In a more recent classification, the preceding phases are together defined as 'early' or 'exploratory' clinical drug development. The corresponding 'late' or 'confirmatory' clinical development phase is then corresponding to the classic phases 2b, 3 and 4. The main objective of phase 2b is proper dose (regimen) finding in hundreds of patients with the targeted disease, whereas phase 3 clinical trials aim at confirming a positive clinical benefit/risk balance versus existing therapies in thousands of patients. If successful after this phase, a marketing authorisation application is filed, allowing the drug, if granted, to be put on the market and generate return on investment. This part of the late development phase is also called the preauthorisation or preapproval phase. Finally, in phase 4 of clinical drug development (the post-authorisation or post-approval phase), the use of the drug in everyday clinical practice is studied, its pharmacovigilance (adverse drug reactions) is (are) monitored and new developments are initiated (for new indications, new associations, or new formulations).

Clinical drug development also involves many different disciplines, each offering several job opportunities. Within clinical drug development organisations (e.g. pharmaceutical companies and CROs), they are usually grouped in the following departments: Clinical Research, Clinical Operations, Medical Review and Pharmacovigilance, Clinical Biometry and Clinical Services, although names can vary from company to company. Their role is to extensively collaborate with one another and generate all clinical data for the marketing authorisation application (preapproval phase), as well as all clinical data for continued developments in the post-approval phase.

Clinical Research is responsible for the content of the clinical development plan of the new drug. They define the strategy, do the planning, oversee the methodology and coordinate the overall (worldwide) management of all clinical trials. In the early clinical development phase, they primarily need clinical pharmacologists, clinical pharmacokineticists, clinical pharmacometricians, but also clinicians (either medical specialists or general practitioners). In the late clinical development phase, this need shifts more towards clinicians and pharmaceutical physicians, pharmaco-epidemiologists and (hospital or clinical) pharmacists.

Clinical Operations is in charge of the implementation of the clinical development plan, the local project management, as well as the monitoring and administration of all clinical trials. They typically hire international and local clinical trial managers, clinical research associates (CRAs or monitors) and clinical trial administrators (CTAs), often with just a master's degree in life sciences (e.g. biomedical or pharmaceutical scientists, research nurses, physiotherapists, or even physicians).

The *Medical Review and Pharmacovigilance* Department is populated by medical reviewers and pharmacovigilance (PV) experts, responsible for the critical review of all medical data gathered in clinical trials and especially all data on adverse events and adverse drug reactions. These aspects are best handled by (pharmaceutical) physicians (hospital or clinical) pharmacists and clinical toxicologists, with the external help of clinicians and medical specialists for specific problems.

The *Clinical Biometry* unit, in charge of clinical data management and clinical statistics, is particularly looking for clinical trial methodologists, data managers, (big) data analysts, biostatisticians and computer programmers.

And finally, the *Clinical Services* Department is responsible for the supply and logistics of all clinical study material, e.g. supply, storage and shipment of investigational drugs (including placebo and comparators) and central laboratory materials (to and fro the study centres, all over the world), or provision of standardised study equipment (e.g. a treadmill for exercise tolerance tests, including the software to run the test). They usually hire pharmaceutical or biomedical scientists for these jobs.

Clinical drug development specialists are also needed in (inter-)national medicines agencies as assessors of the clinical parts of clinical trial or investigational new drug applications (CTA in Europe, IND in USA) and Marketing Authorisation (MA, Europe) or New Drug Applications (NDA, USA).

A particular characteristic of clinical drug development is that clinical trials are largely performed in investigational sites that do not belong to the drug development organisation itself. With the notable exception of phase 1 trials, usually performed in phase 1 units with healthy volunteers (of which some are owned by pharmaceutical companies or CROs), clinical trials recruit patients who can only be found in institutions, e.g. (university) hospitals, academic phase 1 units, or nursing homes, or else in private practices of general practitioners or medical specialists. Besides, many (academic) hospitals perform their own clinical (drug) research as investigator-initiated trials (IIT). All these investigational sites also offer a lot of job opportunities as investigator, research physician, research nurse, study coordinator and clinical research pharmacist. Some sites are grouped in site management organizations (SMO) or specific organizations such as the European Organisation for Research and Treatment of Cancer (EORTC) that coordinate clinical trials for their member sites. They too need qualified professionals.

4.4. Commercialisation

The last part of the drug life cycle and hopefully the longest for many years, is the commercialisation phase. It starts with the marketing authorisation of the new medicine and ends with its withdrawal from the market, thus also ending its life cycle (see **Figure 1**). During this phase, there is a period that an innovative drug can be on the market without competition thanks to its patent protection and additional exclusivity rights, so that the owner can maximise its return of investment (ROI). Once off-patent, sales in general suddenly drop (the patent cliff) because of the introduction of generics or biosimilars, but may find a new equilibrium for years thereafter.

Drug commercialisation activities are mostly the prerogative of pharmaceutical companies, although some can also be subcontracted to CROs. They can be found in the following departments: market access, marketing, medical affairs, production and distribution and sales.

A marketing authorisation is not sufficient to get a drug for human use on the market. You also need to negotiate a fair price with different national health authorities (price setting) and to demonstrate added value in order to gain acceptable coverage or reimbursement conditions with different national health insurance system providers. These steps are known as market access hurdles. *Market access* departments mainly group financial experts, drug pricing specialist, experts in health technology assessment (HTA), pharmaco-economists, core value dossier writers and pharmaceutical policy experts, together with marketing specialists. They generally hire professionals with specific qualifications such as Master of Finance or Economics, but also life scientists (pharmacists, physicians and biomedical scientists) often with a second degree in, for instance, health economics or pharmaceutical medicine. Similar jobs can, of course, also be found in the national institutes, agencies, or committees that have to decide on drug prices and reimbursement conditions.

Pharmaceutical marketing is responsible for promoting the sales of a (new) medicine. It supposes a good knowledge of the pharmaceutical market, general marketing principles (communicating the value of a product to customers), specific pharmaceutical marketing principles (e.g. operating in a regulated market), as well as the specificities of pharmaceutical marketing activities (market analysis, marketing strategy and plan, marketing channels and tools) adapted to the different phases of the commercial life span of a drug (prelaunch, launch, ascending phase, maturity and end-stage phase); and all this, within the rules of local drug promotion, legislation and regulation. This is typically the work space of national or international product managers and brand or group product managers (responsible for several drugs within a given therapeutic area), either specialists with a marketing degree or life scientists with a Master in Business Administration (MBA).

Medical affairs focuses on clinical drug development in the post-approval phase and on the medical and scientific aspects of pharmaceutical marketing, such as managing medical communications and publications, key opinion leaders (KOLs) and advisory boards and medical information (answering questions from health care providers and patients). Medical affairs professionals bridge the gap between R&D and marketing and hold positions such as medical advisor, medical science liaison (MSL), medical information manager, or pharmacovigilance expert, usually filled by physicians or pharmacists, often with a postgraduate degree in pharmaceutical medicine.

Pharmaceutical sales is the ultimate activity that brings in the money to reinvest in new drug R&D. The sales teams are made up of pharmaceutical sales representatives or (medical) reps, who promote (a selection of) the drugs of a pharmaceutical company. Prescription drugs are promoted toward physicians, while non-prescription drugs (over-the-counter or OTC medication) is promoted toward pharmacists. Sales reps are usually responsible for a given franchise or therapeutic class of drugs, a given target audience (private practices or hospitals) and a given local territory. There work is supervised by regional and country sales managers. Most pharmaceutical companies have their own sales force, but additional sales reps can either be (temporarily) insourced from a CRO, or the entire sales activity for a given franchise or brand can be outsourced to a CRO. Sales departments typically hire holders of bachelors and masters in life sciences (including physiotherapists), with strong communication skills and the necessary motivation and stamina to reach sales objectives, which are trained in-house and on the job.

Finally, *pharmaceutical production* facilities make sure that the necessary volumes of medicines are manufactured in due time with high quality, from the active pharmaceutical ingredient (API) to the end product. The *distribution* department sees to it that drug orders are channelled appropriately in order to reach wholesalers, community and hospital pharmacies on a regular basis. This is typically a world of chemical engineers, industrial pharmacists and supply chain managers.

5. Job opportunities in support and management functions

Within drug development organisations (e.g. mostly pharmaceutical companies, CROs or specialised start-ups and more rarely academic research centres or spin-offs), all the disciplines described above have to work together with the additional help of data managers, data analysts, (bio-)statisticians, quality management experts, specialists in regulatory sciences/

affairs, report writers and planning specialists. The coordination and oversight are kept by project team leaders (who prepare the documents needed for decision-making), while go/no go-decisions are taken by (a team of) senior managers.

These activities in the pharma sector are not only important in a specific part of the drug life cycle, but cover the entire business and value chain. They too offer many job opportunities.

5.1. Regulatory sciences/affairs

As the pharmaceutical sector is highly regulated, the regulatory affairs department makes sure that their pharmaceutical organisation or company complies with all (inter-)national legislations, regulations and guidelines pertaining to their business (worldwide). They are at the forefront in the negotiations with medicines agencies when asking them for scientific advice, or when discussing with them about the marketing authorisation of a new drug, or when arguing about changes to the Summary of Product Characteristics of a drug (SmPC in Europe, labelling in USA). They also see to it that all regulatory documents, such as clinical trial applications, marketing authorisation applications and variations, as well as drug safety reports are prepared, assembled and send to the appropriate health authorities in due time. Regulatory affairs professionals may be responsible for a country or a geographical region (e.g. Europe, USA, or Asia), or they may be specialised in preapproval or post-approval affairs. Most of them are pharmacists or occasionally other life scientists, often with a post-graduate in regulatory sciences or pharmaceutical medicine.

5.2. Quality management

The quality of all the activities at all the steps and levels throughout the drug life cycle is assured by a quality management system (QMS) that typically consists of a set of rules and regulations (good practices or GxP), translated into standard operational procedures (SOP), the proper application of which is regularly monitored by quality control during operations (by self-control and monitoring) and occasionally checked by audits (by internal or external auditors) and inspections (by regulatory authorities).

Quality management professionals oversee that all operational departments comply with the recommended best practices, e.g. good laboratory practices (GLP), good clinical practices (GCP), good manufacturing practices (GMP), good pharmacovigilance practices (GVP), good distribution practices (GDP). Typical quality assurance (QA) activities include SOP writing, training of operational staff and investigator teams in quality management and performing audits from which lessons can be learned for further improvement of activities or processes.

QA professionals are usually life scientists, often with a postgraduate degree in quality management and with previous experience in an operational function in the pharmaceutical sector. Inspectors from health authorities are usually pharmacists.

5.3. Scientific/medical writing

All the activities throughout the drug life cycle generate a lot of study reports, publications, regulatory documents and applications to be written in several languages. Most pharma companies have a scientific and/or medical writing department responsible for that. These departments are populated by life scientists and translators with excellent writing and communication skills. Some of these professionals are self-employed and work as external service providers on a freelance basis.

5.4. Training and development (personal, professional)

Most pharmaceutical companies have their proper training department or corporate training academy, but there is also a plethora of training opportunities offered by specialised service providers (either in-house or external). Their objective is to provide the induction training to newcomers (including company-specific strategic thinking and knowledge transfer), as well as continuous training and development for all (individuals and teams). Training activities are offered to all operational disciplines throughout the drug life cycle, e.g. to researchers, clinical research associates, project and product managers and sales reps. These learning activities are not only meant to optimise their technical knowledge, but also target as much at the development of their core workplace skills. Trainers come in all shapes and sizes, have different backgrounds and qualifications, should have some expertise in the field to be taught, but most of all should have excellent communication and teaching abilities and should love to work with people. The rest can be learned on the job by training the trainer.

5.5. Management

The success of any business depends heavily on the effectiveness of its managers. This is equally true in the complex pharmaceutical sector, where many aspects of management come into play, such as strategic management (e.g. innovation, portfolio or risk management and go/no go decision-making) as well as operational management (e.g. project management, clinical, or sales operations). Therefore, there is a high need for visionary leaders and talented managers in this sector. Some people have inborn leadership and management talents, but others grow in it during their career development. Senior and corporate managers in the pharmaceutical business have different backgrounds and qualifications, from life scientists to economists and lawyers, often with a Master in Business Administration (MBA).

6. Career perspectives

At entry, young professionals are often employed as a junior or an assistant, preceding their functional job title (e.g. Junior or Assistant Project Manager). After a year or two, these prefixes can be dropped and after an additional number of years of experience in the same job the prefix can change to Senior (e.g. Senior Project Manager).

Initial on-the-job training and work experience can be gained during traineeships, internships, job or work shadowing, secondments and temp jobs (all paid or not).

In the (bio-)pharmaceutical industry, many young academics start their career as an employee of a CRO, which then outsources them for a certain period (6 months or a year) to a pharmaceutical company for a specific job. After a couple of such secondments in different companies, these young professionals get a better idea of what they really want and what is offered out there for their future career development.

After an initial work experience of a varying number of years, young professionals usually start thinking of their career development in the pharmaceutical sector. An important element to consider is whether you want to stay an expert in your field or become a manager or a leader, as they require different skills, training and work experience.

Career moves can be of several types:

- You can move along the path of the drug life cycle, e.g. you can start in Clinical Operations (as Project Manager) and move to Regulatory Affairs (as Country or Regional Manager) or Marketing (as Product Manager). Moving backwards from marketing to R&D is much harder though.

- You can move lateral (e.g. switch in the same position from one country to another) or move up (e.g. become a Project Team Manager or Group Product Manager).

- You can start an international career, working in several countries worldwide and then return to the company headquarters for a senior management job.

- You can switch from one company to another within the pharmaceutical industry, or you can switch from a CRO to a pharma company, or you can switch back to academia, or start a career in a governmental agency.

With every career move, you confront new challenges and over the years you get more responsibility, eventually as senior manager. The ultimate move may be that you become Chief Executive Officer (CEO), the 'big boss' of a company.

As an alternative career option, you can also start your own company, either as a young entrepreneur or as a senior consultant. Both these options require a solid business plan and an entrepreneurial mindset.

7. Training opportunities

Given the high number of job and career opportunities described above, the main challenge for young students and graduates is to understand which are their preferred jobs and how to get them.

A useful approach is to attend all possible orientation events such as career days, organised nowadays by most universities in which it is possible to listen to experts coming from different companies.

Some of the biggest pharmaceutical companies, including Abbott[1], AbbVie[2], Amgen[3], Astra-Zeneca[4], Baxter[5], Bayer[6], Biogen[7], Boehringer-Ingelheim[8], Bristol-Myers Squibb[9], Eli Lilly & Co[10], Gilead[11], GlaxoSmithKline[12], Johnson & Johnson[13], Merck & Co[14], Merck KGaA[15], Novartis[16], Novo

Nordisk [17], Roche [18], Sanofi [19], Teva [20] have excellent traineeship programmes for young students and graduates.

Useful websites to find excellent scientific positions in public or private institutions are https://www.sciencemag.org/careers, http://www.nature.com/naturejobs/science/, http://jobs.newscientist.com/, etc.

Another valuable strategy is to apply for a traineeship in a company in another European country participating in the Erasmus+ programme.[21] The programme offers the possibility of spending periods of at least two months in non-academic institutions including pharmaceutical companies and research centres.[22] Most universities are active in this programme and students can easily obtain detailed information from their international offices.

Some European Institutions such as the European Medicines Agency (EMA),[23] the European Centre for Disease Prevention and Control (ECDC),[24] and the European Patent Office (EPO)[25] offer very interesting traineeships.

---

[1] http://www.abbott.com/careers/students/development-programs.html

[2] http://www.abbvie.com/careers/student-opportunities/development-programs.html

[3] http://careers.amgen.com/university-relations/internships-co-ops/

[4] http://www.astrazenecacareers.com/students/programmes/

[5] http://www.baxter.com/careers/programs/healthcare-internships-co-ops.page

[6] https://career.bayer.com/en/career/working-at-bayer/students/

[7] https://www.biogen-international.com/en/careers1/pharmd-fellowships.html

[8] http://careers.boehringer-ingelheim.com/students

[9] http://www.bms.com/careers/university_recruitment/internships_co-ops/pages/graduates_undergraduates.aspx

[10] https://careers.lilly.com/campus

[11] http://www.gilead.com/careers/careers/current-opportunities

[12] http://futureleaders.gsk.com/en-gb/our-programmes/

[13] http://www.careers.jnj.com/explore-careers-student

[14] http://www.merck.com/careers/life-at-merck/students-and-graduates.html

[15] http://www.merckgroup.com/en/careers/graduates_and_students/faq/faq.html

[16] https://www.novartis.com/careers

[17] http://www.novonordisk.com/careers/graduates-students-and-trainees/graduates/graduate-programmes-overview-uk.html

[18] http://www.roche.com/careers/switzerland/ch_your_job/students_and_graduates/trainee_programs.htm

[19] http://en.sanofi.com/careers/join_sanofi/graduates_interns/graduates_interns.aspx

[20] http://www.tevapharm.com/tova_careers/european_leadership_programme/

[21] https://ec.europa.eu/programmes/erasmus-plus/node_en

[22] https://ec.europa.eu/programmes/erasmus-plus/individuals_en#tab-1-4

[23] http://www.ema.europa.eu/ema/index.jsp?curl=pages/about_us/general/general_content_000321.jsp

[24] http://ecdc.europa.eu/en/aboutus/jobs/Pages/Traineeships.aspx

[25] http://www.epo.org/about-us/jobs/vacancies/internships.html

The Innovative Medicine Initiative (IMI),[26] Europe's largest public-private initiative aiming to speed up the development of better and safer medicines for patients, has several interesting projects in the field of education and training:

- European Medicines Research Training Network[27] (EMTRAIN), a platform for education and training covering the whole life cycle of medicines research, from basic science through clinical development to pharmacovigilance.

- European programme in Pharmacovigilance and Pharmacoepidemiology[28] (Eu2P) which developed numerous courses covering various aspects of medicines' research and development, including pharmacovigilance.

- Pharmaceutical Medicine Training Programme[29] (Pharmatrain), which established standards for high-quality postgraduate education and training in Medicines Development.

- European Modular Education and Training Programme in Safety Sciences for Medicines[30] (SafeSciMET) which established a new and unique pan-European education and training network, providing master's level courses in safety sciences for medicines.

Another important question often asked by students and graduates is related to the necessary level of education required for the different positions in the pharmaceutical sector. The answer to it is not always easy because despite the harmonization of the architecture of the European higher education obtained through the Bologna process since 1999[31] (1st cycle or bachelor's degree, 2nd cycle or master's degree, 3rd cycle or PhD or Doctorate), there are still significant differences in the pharmaceutical field. In most European countries, while chemistry, biology and biotechnology are usually studied in two subsequent cycles (bachelor + master), pharmacy and industrial pharmacy are usually 5 or 6 years integrated master's degree programmes. In addition, in some countries, such as Italy and France for example, it is very common to attend a 'professional master' after the master's degree to obtain the necessary knowledge and skills to be hired by pharma companies for positions in clinical monitoring, pharmacovigilance, or regulatory affairs. Finally, concerning the third cycle, despite the existence of many different research and professional PhDs, it should be mentioned that in most countries, the title of PhD is really necessary for careers in research, but not for most of the other positions described in this chapter.

---

[26] http://www.imi.europa.eu/

[27] http://www.emtrain.eu/

[28] https://www.eu2p.org/

[29] http://www.pharmatrain.eu/

[30] http://www.safescimet.eu/

[31] http://ec.europa.eu/education/policy/higher-education/bologna-process_en.htm

8. Important employability elements

8.1. Wanted qualifications

Apart from technical qualifications, it is important to develop managerial leadership competences. So how do we know what leadership competences are important to career success? The Association to Advance Collegiate Schools of Business (AACSB) [2], which gives accreditation to business schools, developed a list of "General Skills Areas" that students are expected to develop:

- Written and oral communication: able to communicate effectively orally and in writing.

- Ethical understanding and reasoning: able to identify ethical issues and address the issues in a socially responsible manner.

- Analytical thinking: able to analyse and frame problems.

- Information technology: able to use current technologies in business and management contexts.

- Interpersonal relations and teamwork: able to work effectively with others and in a team environment.

- Diverse and multicultural work environments: able to work effectively in diverse environments.

- Reflective thinking: able to understand oneself in the context of society.

- Application of knowledge: able to translate knowledge into practice.

8.2. Vitae employability lens

Vitae is a non-profit organisation based in Cambridge, UK, with almost 50 years of experience in enhancing the skills and careers of researchers. As a spin-off of these activities, Vitae has developed an Employability Lens that could serve as a researcher development framework for careers outside academia. This tool gives an overview of the key knowledge, behaviours and attributes that are typically important for graduates from academia and as such often appreciated by employers, see link to the pdf below:

https://www.vitae.ac.uk/vitae-publications/rdf-related/employability-lens-vitae-researcher-development-framework-rdf-may-2012.pdf

The Vitae Employability Lens is particularly useful in identifying additional skills on top of the specific key knowledge of academics seeking employment outside academia, for example, in the drug development field. To achieve this, it especially focuses on behaviours and attitudes, rather than on the knowledge base that has been the original aim of studies and training during academic studies. In doing so, the lens can serve as an 'eye opener' especially for PhD holders that primarily expected to valorise their theoretical knowledge and their technical experience. Thanks to this employability lens, a range of transferable skills has been identified that has proved to be added value in almost any workplace, thereby significantly lowering the threshold for academic graduates to make the step towards industry. In addition, these transferable skills can be trained and many Doctoral Schools provide focused short training programs as a way to effectively support the career perspectives of PhD researchers after obtaining their degree.

Apart from this focus on transferable skills, it can be expected that many academically trained researchers will wonder in what part of the drug life cycle their specific knowledge base could still provide an added value. This would enable them to valorise their specific knowledge and experience and thus provide a basis for a career after making the step from academia towards the pharmaceutical sector. An overview of specific knowledge needed in the Drug Life Cycle is given below in **Table 1**.

Academic knowledge base for employment		Drug life cycle expressed in five stages:				
Academic fields by discipline	Academic degree	Research discovery & design	Non-clinical development	Early clinical development	Late clinical development	Commercialisation
Pharmaceutical sciences	MA		×		×	×
Pharmaceutical sciences	PhD	××	××	×		
Medical sciences	MD			×	×	×
Medical sciences	MD-PhD	××	×	××	×	
Biomedical sciences	MA				×	×
Biomedical sciences	PhD	××	××			
Veterinary sciences	MA	×	×			
Veterinary sciences	PhD	××	××			
Pharmacy	MA		×	×	×	
Pharmacy	PhD	××	××			
Industrial pharmacy	MA		×	×	×	×
Industrial pharmacy	PhD	××	××			

Academic knowledge base for employment		Drug life cycle expressed in five stages:				
Academic fields by discipline	Academic degree	Research discovery & design	Non-clinical development	Early clinical development	Late clinical development	Commercialisation
Biotechnologies	MA		×		×	×
Biotechnologies	PhD	××	××			
Chemistry	MA		×			
Chemistry	PhD	××	××			
Biology	MA					
Biology	PhD	××	××			
Biochemistry	MA					
Biochemistry	PhD	×	××			
Physics	MA					
Physics	PhD	×	×			
(Bio)informatics	MA	×	×			
(Bio)informatics	PhD	××	×			
Engineering	MA		×			×
Engineering	PhD	×	×	×	×	
Mathematics and data analysis	MA/PhD	×	×	×	×	
Law and legal studies	MA	×	×	×	×	××
Economy and finance	MA					×
Business administration	MA (MBA)					×
Communication studies	MA/PhD				×	×
Languages	MA				×	×

Table 1. Overview of specific knowledge needed in the drug life cycle.

In **Table 1**, the academic knowledge base for employment has been linked to the various stages of the drug life cycle, as introduced in the beginning of this chapter. The clinical development stage has just been divided into two phases (early and late), followed by the commercialisation stage after marketing authorisation. The aim of **Table 1** is to document that disciplinary knowledge is also very important in the drug development process and that different disciplines contribute to different stages of the drug life cycle. Combined studies are not indicated in **Table 1**, but can be quite valuable, for example, a primary degree in Pharmaceutical Sciences and a second degree in Patent Law.

As can be seen in **Table 1**, the most important academic knowledge base is contributed by PhD holders in the various molecular, biotech and life sciences during stages 1 and 2, which are focused on drug discovery and non-clinical development. Academics with a background in the pharmaceutical and medical sciences can typically use their knowledge base during the whole drug life cycle. For the more advanced stages in the life cycle, a PhD could still be an advantage, but the valorisation of academic knowledge developed during the PhD studies will likely become less important, while the transferable skills and behaviours of PhD holders will start to predominate. This also implies that a vast range of academics listed in **Table 1**, can professionally contribute to any of the stages of the drug life cycle. The fact that crosses are lacking in certain positions merely indicates that in those positions the original academic knowledge base is unlikely to be the main contributor to the activities in that stage. Thus, a biologist that is employed as a Clinical Research Associate (CRA) and active in the later stage of clinical development will not have a cross in this part of **Table 1** (because there is no dominance of biological key knowledge in that stage), but he/she can still build out a very interesting career. **Table 1** is not based on quantitative data but rather reflects the authors' views on where specific academic disciplinary knowledge is expected to be most valuable in the drug life cycle.

9. Effective job application

9.1. Introduction

Successful job application requires three things: (1) having a good motivation, (2) having the required technical skill set and (3) being able to illustrate your interpersonal skills.

Having a good motivation concerns three levels, motivation for the content of the job (*what do you think this job entails on a daily basis?*), motivation for the organisation (*why do you want to work for us?*) and being able to express your own professional goals (*where do you want to be in 3 years?*). These three should line up. Desirably one's own professional goals are in line with the mission of the organisation.

Having the required technical skill set. Technical skills involve the ability to use methods and techniques to perform a task. Employers are looking for a candidate with a specific specialisation or specific degree or a previous work experience in a specific field of activity (R&D, marketing, sales, etc.) and sector. They want to be convinced that new employees will be able to do the job content wise.

For example QA professionals are usually life scientists, often with a postgraduate degree in quality management and with previous experience in an operational function in the pharmaceutical sector.

Being able to illustrate your interpersonal skills. Interpersonal skills involve to the ability to understand, communicate and work well with individuals and groups through developing effective relationships. Employers often refer to this as having the 'right attitude'. They want to learn about the candidates' positive and negative sides and how they cope with difficult situations at work, for example, *how do you solve problems or deal with conflicts*? Employers want to avoid hiring staff that are not a good match with the team. Employers will verify this by asking questions with regard to soft skills (*what is your role in a team, tell us a bit more about your communication skills, we are looking for somebody with proven leadership skills, etc.*).

9.2. Tips and tricks for a cover letter

The cover letter functions to express motivation and qualifications for the job.

- It is important to be concise and not too long (not more than one A4-page).

- Make an overview of the required hard and soft skills of the job advertisement.

- As a recent graduate you may not have all the required skills. You can still apply when covering 70–80% of all skills required.

- Make sure that the cover letter mentions all the hard and soft skills that you have.

- Use as much as possible the labels that are used in the job advertisement.

- With regard to the soft skills: describe a few activities in your current work or projects that illustrate your roles and results.

- Make clear what is important to you in your work (your professional goals) and how this links to the job content and the goals of the organization.

- Highlight those qualifications that make you an outstanding candidate.

- Use strong wording (not I think or I believe) and don't make interpretations for the jury.

9.3. Tips and tricks for a curriculum vitae (CV) or resume

- Again employers look for motivation and skills, make sure that you illustrate both in your CV.

- The work experience section is most important, describe all your roles and quantify the results. Also include relevant extracurricular activities and internships.

- You may include your motivation by adding a short elevator pitch (*summary/professional goals*) in your personal data section at the beginning of your CV. By doing so, employers know what you are heading for.

- Your CV should be in line with your LinkedIn profile and other open sources available on the Internet with regard to your profile (Twitter, Facebook, Research gate, etc.).

- Be short and concise (max. two A4-pages).

9.4. Tips and tricks for a job interview

- The purpose of a job interview is to sell yourself and receive a job offer.

- A job interview starts with introducing yourself: prepare an elevator pitch.

- With regard to motivation: formulate what you can add to the organisation, not what is in it for yourself.

- Your body language is very important. Talk slowly, look into the eyes of all the jury members, give a firm handshake and have a confident look.

- Stay cool during a job interview; do not get irritated, even if the jury asks you confronting questions.

- Prepare three examples of your biggest achievements in your work, studies, or extracurricular activities that you can use to illustrate your skills. Describe the context, your role, the activities that you initiated and the results.

- Make sure that you can reflect on your results. Employers love employees who are open for criticism and want to improve continuously.

- Prepare three positive sides and three negative sides. Explain how you cope with your downsides.

- Many tricky questions are another way of checking again on your motivation and qualifications for the job. Just repeat what you have been saying in a nice way.

- Never discuss money or benefits before you are offered a job.

10. Conclusion

Our writing of this chapter is based on the notion that a successful launch of a career in the pharmaceutical sector depends on an overall knowledge of this sector and on a smart strategy for job application. Besides these two key elements, many companies recruit via their traineeship programs as discussed in Section 7. One should realise that also in this sector, the vast majority of jobs are never advertised. For this reason, training and networking is indeed a far more effective job-seeking strategy than screening magazines and websites for advertisements. This partly hidden job market also implies that the first step from academia to the pharmaceutical sector is often experienced as the hardest and most important one; it will determine your direction and your differentiation as an employee. At the same time, you will access a new network of professionals with its own word-of-mouth that can become vital for your next career moves.

Besides all the aspects already treated in this chapter, there are only a few closing remarks left, worth to take into account. Jobs in the pharmaceutical sector often come in location-related clusters in Europe. These so-called research parks are often located near international research-oriented universities, where graduates are directly available for recruitment purposes. When new centres are opened, often several jobs are available, even if you can only apply for one at the time. One should realise that these new centres could only become successful when the vacancies are rapidly filled and the industrial annual targets are reached in that specific location. If vacancies stay open too long, the company will most likely move to another location. This implies that research and development hot spots in, for example, Europe can compete with each other through the speed they reach in filling their vacancies and grow more successful as a site. For this reason, it is very important for academic graduates with the right qualifications to be willing to move to a new national or international location, to fill that vacancy that perfectly matches their particular hard and soft skills and become employed in a larger R&D hotspot that might also offer perspectives for additional career moves in the future. It requires some additional study and networking to become aware of the upcoming hotspots relevant for your particular area of interest.

A last reflection is about the important work versus private life balance. If you talk to successful people in the pharmaceutical sector, you will often quickly discover that they really love their job and that, as a consequence, they work a lot. This does not mean that they have squeezed their family life to a minimum, but there are positions in this sector that simply demand more than just the regular office hours. Companies may differ in their philosophies about the work-life and gender balance and it can be an advantage to know their general view about this.

Further improvement of human health largely depends on the development of new methods in prevention, early diagnosis and treatment of disease. An input of new knowledge from young employees with fresh inspiration and energy to achieve this goal is vital for the pharmaceutical sector. With this chapter, we hope to have opened the door and lowered the threshold to enter an exciting world of opportunities.

Author details

Josse R. Thomas[1], Chris van Schravendijk[2], Lucia Smit[3] and Luciano Saso[4*]

*Address all correspondence to: luciano.saso@uniroma1.it

1 Faculty of Pharmaceutical Sciences, KU Leuven, Leuven, Belgium

2 Faculty of Medicine and Pharmacy, Vrije Universiteit Brussel, Brussels, Belgium

3 Braingain, Empowering Young Professionals, Brussels, Belgium

4 Faculty of Pharmacy and Medicine, Sapienza University of Rome, Rome, Italy

References

[1] Rosier JA, Martens MA, Thomas JR. Global New Drug Development: An Introduction, Wiley Blackwell, John Wiley & Sons Ltd., UK: 2014

[2] AACSB website (htpp://www.aacsb.edu/accreditation/standards) in: Leadership: Theory, Application & Skill Development, 6th edition, Lussier, R.N., Achua, C.F., Cengage Learning, USA: 2016.

5

Schistosomiasis: Setting Routes for Drug Discovery

Naiara Clemente Tavares,

Pedro Henrique Nascimento de Aguiar,

Sandra Grossi Gava, Guilherme Oliveira and

Marina Moraes Mourão

Additional information is available at the end of the chapter

Abstract

Schistosomiasis is the second most prevalent parasitic disease in the world. Currently, the treatment of this disease relies on a single drug, praziquantel, and due to the identification of resistant parasites, the development of new drugs is urged. The demand for the development of robust high-throughput parasite screening techniques is increasing as drug discovery research in schistosomiasis gains significance. Here, we review the most common methods used for compound screening in the parasites life stages and also summarize some of the methods that have been recently developed. In addition, we reviewed the methods most commonly implemented to search for promising targets and how they have been used to validate new targets against the parasite *Schistosoma mansoni*. We also review some promising targets in this parasite and show the main approaches and the major advances that have been achieved by those studies. Moreover, we share our experiences in schistosomiasis drug discovery attained with our *S. mansoni* drug screening platform establishment.

Keywords: *Schistosoma mansoni*, drug screening, histone-modifying enzymes, protein kinases, inhibitors, RNA interference

1. Introduction

Schistosomiasis is a chronic parasitic disease caused by flatworms of the genus *Schistosoma*. The main species of medical relevance are *Schistosoma mansoni*, *Schistosoma japonicum*, and *Schistosoma haematobium*, which infect around 258 million people worldwide, causing 300,000 deaths yearly, according to WHO statistics. The economic and health effects of schistosomiasis are considerable as this disease can be highly debilitating. To date, there is no licensed vaccine against the disease, and treatment is based on a single drug, praziquantel [1, 2]. Despite its effectiveness, the heavy reliance on a single drug bears a risk of drug resistance development and, indeed, resistant parasites have already been reported [3–7]. Additionally, praziquantel presents poor efficacy against immature schistosome life stage, and there is no pediatric formulation available. Hence, drug discovery in schistosomiasis is still of great importance.

2. Drug screening techniques in schistosomiasis

Several approaches are used to search new drugs for infectious diseases. Among them, we can highlight: selective, empirical, biochemical, and genomic approaches. In the selective approach, compounds targeting molecules important for parasite survival and/or development (a "chokepoint") are tested. The empirical method consists of a blind random test of a large number of compounds, without any previous knowledge. The biochemical approach verifies whether the compounds are capable to change parasite metabolism. Finally, the genomic approach aims to search for new drug targets based on parasite and/or host genome analysis [8, 9].

Drug screening in *Schistosoma* has been performed using a myriad of techniques and, most of the time, using a single life stage. In order to optimize drug screening in a parasite presenting such distinct and complex life cycle, the search for inhibitors must be performed in the different human infecting life cycle stages such as the schistosomula and adult worms (males and females) as drug sensitivity can differ between the stages and sexes [7]. The screening should also be conducted *in vitro* and *in vivo* since drug activity can be diverse in different systems.

A wide range of *in vitro* methods for drug screening in *S. mansoni* is described; however, microscopic observation to identify the presence of intracellular granularity and changes in the shape and movement of the parasite remains the most used technique, and it is considered the "gold standard" for parasite viability evaluation [10, 11]. However, this analysis can be subjective: (1) it relies in one observing person; (2) schistosomula may exhibit characteristics of dead specimens even when viable [12]; and (3) it is time consuming.

Recently, new methods based on high-throughput (HTS) and whole-organism screens in helminths have emerged. The HTS method is based on screening a parasite target against a large number of compounds in parallel (minimum of 10,000) and may be performed manually or automatically using robotic systems [13–15]. In contrast, the whole-organism screen intends to test a small number of compounds against the pathogen and the drug effect is usually individually analyzed [16]. These new methods monitor the parasite by video, impedance, enzymatic activity, colorimetry, and fluorimetry among others [17–23].

An example of fluorimetric method is the quantification of lactate excreted by the parasite in the culture medium. The parasite tegument presents two glucose transporters, SGTP1 and SGTP4, which acquire glucose present in the host bloodstream [24]. Lactate is the final product after glycolysis, and it is excreted through aquaporin SmAQP, an aquaglyceroporin homologue [25]. The amount of lactate excreted by the parasite can be measured by fluorimetric assays with probes that bind to lactate and emit fluorescence. The measurement of lactate produced by cells has frequently been used for the analysis of cells or whole-organism viability [26, 27]. This method was used by Howe and collaborators [17] and was proved feasible in *S. mansoni*, owing to its sensitivity to measure the viability of adult worms and schistosomula.

Fluorescence viability analysis in schistosomula was also performed by Peak and collaborators [23] combining the use of propidium iodide (PI) (544 nm excitation/620 nm emission) and fluorescein diacetate (FDA) (485 nm excitation/520 nm emission). The PI intercalates into DNA if the membrane of cells is permeable in damaged or dead parasites, but in viable schistosomula, PI is incapable to cross the membrane. Breach of the membrane permeability allows PI to stain nucleic acids. On the other hand, FDA is able to penetrate the membrane of live schistosomula, and due to the parasite esterase activity, it is converted into a highly fluorescent and charged fluorescein, and FDA cannot readily exit living cells. This test requires a fluorescence inverted microscope to evaluate each spectrum. However, even without a fluorescence readout, staining with PI is a quantitative, simple and low-cost method that has been used for a long time for viability evaluation in *S. mansoni* by our group [28].

The blue dye resazurin has been widely used in drug testing in *Trypanosoma* and *Leishmania* species [29, 30]. This method relies on an oxidation-reduction reaction, wherein resazurin suffers a colorimetric change in response to cellular metabolic reduction. The reduced form is pink, and thus, the intensity of fluorescence produced is proportional to the number of living cells. Despite being described as an effective drug test for *S. mansoni* and demonstrating that they were able to detect schistosomula viability, its use is questionable since, when compared to the visual test, this method showed low sensitivity [22]. In our hands, this method has proven very variable among replicates and requires a very specific fluorescence plate reader.

Movement-based assays are widely used for anthelmintic drug screening in adult worms and might be the first phenotype tested in most screenings, whereas movement measures are not explored as much for testing viability of the *S. mansoni* larval stage. Kotze et al. [31] performed visual assays to test drug sensitivity in *Strongyloides* species. This method consisted in scoring the larvae that exhibited movement after 48 h of drug incubation and stimulation with hot water. The approach proved to be an efficient assay for testing new drugs and for detection of resistance; nevertheless, it is quite subjective. Meanwhile, Paveley et al. [19] performed a phenotype analysis in *S. mansoni* schistosomula exposed to drugs. The authors developed an image-based method that collects images in time-lapse every 6 s and analyzes the cumulative change in the area occupied by each schistosomulum. The researchers concluded that this method is suitable for drug screening in schistosomula, although requiring a complex analysis involving machine training.

Recently, Rinaldi et al. [11] have adapted a cell viability method, which is based on impedance, called xCELLigence, to evaluate the movement of cercariae, schistosomula and adult worms, and measure egg hatching of *S. mansoni*. This assay consists in analyzing the changes in electric conductivity due to parasite contact with electrodes; therefore, more parasite movement is measured as a large electric conductivity change. The possibility of using this method in drug screening using cercariae, adult worms, and eggs was also verified. However, this method is at a preliminary stage of standardization, since only one drug was tested and exhibited large variation across electrical frequencies tested; in addition, the cost of the equipment and its plates is elevated.

A very promising method that provides a viability assay in a high-throughput fashion and with semiquantitative measurements of movement of helminth worms was developed by Marcellino and collaborators [18]. This method has demonstrated to be efficient and sensitive for drug screening using *S. mansoni* adult worms, since worm movement is considered an important parameter for high performance tests. In this assay, a video camera and a free software, called WormAssay, are required and output adult worm movement units. The smaller the value of movement units generated by the software, the lower the parasite viability. Later, this methodology, named it as Worminator, was adapted to be used with microscopic parasites as third-stage larvae of *Cooperia* spp. and *Brugia malayi* and *Dirofilaria immitis* microfilariaes. Therefore, Worminator could be an efficient alternative for measuring schisto-somula motility [32].

Another promising method based on video capture was developed by Lee and collaborators [14]. This assay is an automated method to analyze images of schistosomula or other parasites in 96, 384, or 1536 well plate format and qualify innumerous phenotypes. A machine-trained algorithm was able to quantitatively describe the following characteristics: size, shape, movement, texture, and color. With this method, it is possible to perform a high-throughput whole-organism drug screening. The web server called quantal dose-response calculator (QDREC), which was described by Asarnow and collaborators [33], is based on this method-ology. QDREC compares drug-treated parasites with untreated parasites and automatically determines dose-response. This method is the only automated method to date that provides EC50 (half maximal effective concentration) values based on phenotypic analysis. QDREC was validated using schistosomula and proved to be a high-throughput and reliable method.

For *in vivo* assays, mice are suggested as the animals of choice, owing to their susceptibility to experimental infection [8, 34]. Thus, mice are infected with cercariae and treated with drugs. After infection, one should observe eggs and granuloma numbers in the liver and intestine, oogram alterations, and number of adult worms recovered after perfusion [35]. This method has been employed using single or combination of praziquantel and in association with lovastatin, clonazepam, among others.

3. Case studies

In order to perform *in vivo* assays, mice infected with *S. mansoni* for 45 days were treated with a single dose of imatinib. After 15 days of treatment, the animals were killed and perfused. *In vitro* tests with imatinib impaired movement of adult worms; however, when mice were treated with this drug, no alterations were found in the oogram and adult worm recovery, demon-strating the need of a complete assay during drug screening [36]. In addition, Pereira and collaborators [37] tested the compound (−)-6,6'-dinitrohinokinin (DNK), a dibenzylbutyrolactone lignin, using *in vitro* and *in vivo* assays. This compound seems to affect the development and reproduction of the parasite as it caused reduction in adult worm recovery and significantly decreased egg count, corroborating the results of *in vitro* tests. These findings reaffirm the need for *in vivo* testing to confirm drug efficacy, since the biological effects highly rely on host metabolism.

Drug combinations for infectious diseases therapy represent an alternative to retard drug resistance. Based on that premise, Araújo et al. [38] treated infected mice with a single dose of clonazepam associated with praziquantel or oxamniquine. The results showed alterations in the oogram and a higher number of dead worms recovered from liver of mice treated with both clonazepam and praziquantel, in comparison with mice treated only with praziquantel. In another study, the association of praziquantel and oxamniquine with lovastatin was investigated *in vivo,* and a higher number of dead adult worms, as well as oogram changes, were observed in mice treated with the combination lovastatin and oxamniquine compared to animals treated with praziquantel [38]. These findings suggest that drug combination is a promising alternative for schistosomiasis treatment.

Thus, it is highly relevant to follow systematic procedures during drug screening. Here, we present a schematic workflow of the above-mentioned methods and different life stages that could be included in drug screening experiments (**Figure 1**).

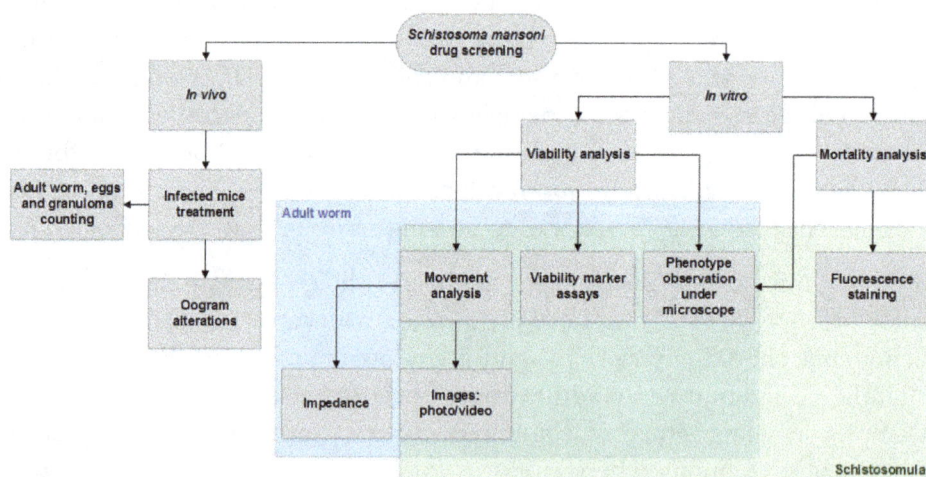

Figure 1. *Schistosoma mansoni* compound screening methods. The workflow represents *in vivo* and *in vitro* assays which can be employed for drug/compounds screening in S. *mansoni*.

4. Establishment of an anti-*Schistosoma mansoni* drug screening platform

The absence of efficient alternative for schistosomiasis treatment demonstrates the need for new research involving the development of new schistosomicidal compounds. Accordingly,

development of a *S. mansoni* drug screening platform, which aims at the study of compound/ drug efficacy in different parasite life stages using distinct methodological approaches is required. To date, our group has immersed in this field seeking new methodologies, standardization of existing ones, and validation of results between different laboratories working in the field. It is important to highlight that *Schistosoma* strains vary in response to treatment, and in order to attain relevant leads, a concerted effort is important. Here we present some data of drug screening in schistosomula and adult worm stages and the comparison of four *in vitro* methodologies.

For drug screening in schistosomula, the methods of choice were: resazurin fluorescence assay, lactate quantitative analysis, and visual assay using propidium iodide staining (PI). In order to perform drug screening in adult worms, the movement analysis software WormAssay was employed.

The standardization for schistosomula drug screening was performed using 96-well plate format with 100, 200, 400, 600, and 800 parasites per well. Schistosomula were submitted to three different treatments: parasites exposed to 0.1% dimethyl sulfoxide (DMSO; vehicle control); heat-killed parasites (negative control); and parasites exposed to 20 μM of the sirtuin inhibitor Salermide (half maximal inhibitory concentration—IC50). Lancelot et al. [39] demonstrated that Salermide induces death and apoptosis of schistosomula, separation of adult worm pairs, as well as a reduction in egg laying.

The PI staining procedure was established by the use of 5 μg/mL of fluorophore into 96-well culture plates containing 100 parasites and visualized in inverted fluorescence microscope. Our results have shown that mortality evaluation by phenotype observation in bright-field light microscope was overestimated when compared to PI staining results. This result reinforces the subjectivity problem of bright-field visual analysis since parasites that presented a dead phenotype (intracellular granularity and absence of movement) not always stain with PI, indicating their viability.

In viability assays using resazurin, we observed large variability between technical and biological replicates and a low value of relative fluorescence units (RFU). Mansour and Bickle [22] described RFU values >1000 in wells containing 100 schistosomula, and such high RFU values were possible only with 500 parasites per well in our assays conditions. Overall, using this fluorescence assay, we were unable to discriminate schistosomula killed by Salermide treatment from the vehicle control (0.1% DMSO). Issues in assay sensitivity measured by RFU values could be due to differences in the fluorescence reader platform, indicating that the assay can present a reproducibility issue. Limitations in this methodology such as low sensitivity and reliability, when compared to visual analysis, were described by the authors who proposed the application of resazurin as *S. mansoni* viability test [22].

Standardization of lactate quantitative analysis demonstrated low variability and significant differences between RFU values of schistosomula exposed to 20 μM Salermide from 0.1% DMSO. RFU values were similar to those described in the work of Howe and collaborators [17] confirming the method's reproducibility. Mortality of the parasites detected in the lactate quantitative analysis was confirmed by PI staining and observation under the microscope, in contrast to our previous results with resazurin assay. Considering the fluorescence-based viability assays, lactate quantitative analysis has shown to be more reliable in our hands. However, the test may also be subject to interference, since some compounds crystallize in contact with culture medium and can emit fluorescence at the wavelength utilized (530 nm excitation/590 nm emission).

The use of viability assays that target schistosome metabolism is important for drug screening, since some drugs may reduce parasite viability but do not cause parasite death, and hence these parasites may not stain by PI. Therefore, we believe that the combination of these two approaches to evaluate parasite viability/mortality is a good strategy for drug screening as they are complementary methodologies.

Regarding adult worm drug screening, Howe and collaborators [17] proposed the use of one male adult worm per well exposed for 72-h treatment with praziquantel and mefloquine, and detected a reduction in medium lactate. The use of only males and one parasite per well does not validate this methodology for drug testing in adult worms, as males and females may react differently to treatments and each individual has distinct susceptibility/metabolism. Therefore, the use of this method would require larger number of worms including both sexes.

The method of trematode movement analysis using impedance was described by Smout and collaborators [20] and was recently validated in *S. mansoni* [11]. In this study, one worm per well was also challenged and wide variation in sensitivity of the experiment was reported due to variation in the electric frequency (kHz). Due to the limitations in those methods, we implemented the WormAssay [18] to analyze adult worm exposure to drugs.

In our platform, eight adult worms were established as the minimum number of specimens to be analyzed. Most importantly, paired females and males should not be analyzed because a drug could be active in only sex, disturbing the movement analysis due to female presence in male gynaecophoric channel. The plates containing the worms are filmed for 1 min and 30 s every day for 10 days. The software is freely available for download, recognizes the wells, and provides the total of movement units for each. Moreover, handling is simple and our tests confirm its sensitivity and accuracy.

For validation of our anti-*S. mansoni* drug screening platform, we used epigenetic modification factor inhibitors. A total of 137 compounds were tested on *S. mansoni* schistosomula and adult worms as part of the A-PARADDISE consortium (http://a-paraddise.cebio.org/) using the visual assay with PI, the quantitative analysis of lactate for schistosomula, and the WormAssay for adult worms. Among these compounds, 114 (83%) exhibited some effect on the parasite. From 114 active compounds, 29 were active in all methods used, and in both sexes and stages tested, 12 compounds were active only in schistosomula, 35 were active at least in one sex of adult worm and, among them, 24 were active only in female worms (**Figure 2**).

These data confirm the need to perform an assay aimed at identifying compounds capable of altering the parasite metabolism and, consequently, their viability, since the compound cannot cause parasite death, hindering the observation of drug effect in a visual assay. Clustering methodologies, life stages, and parasite strains could change the outcomes of large screening studies such as those using a single method and stage; for example, Li et al. [40] performed a screening of 59,360 thioredoxin glutathione reductase (TGR) inhibitors against *S. mansoni* thioredoxin glutathione reductase (SmTGR) recombinant protein using a fluorometric assay, 74 were active and tested in *S. mansoni*, and among them, 53% were active in schistosomula and only 2.7% were effective against adult worms. Additionally, Yousif et al. [41] carried out a screen of 309 plant extracts on adult worms employing visual analysis of viability and identified 14% as active.

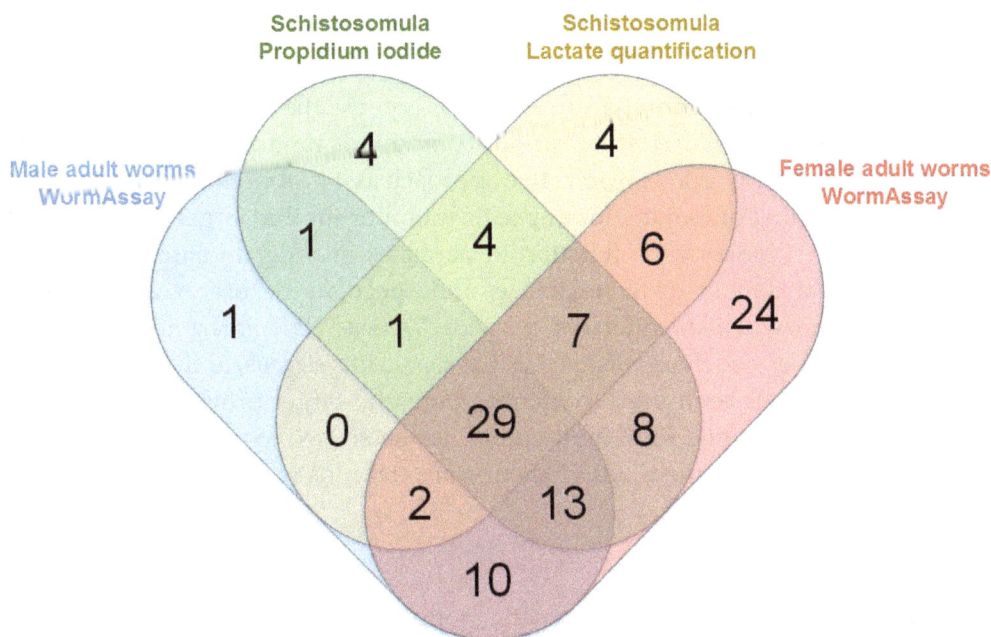

Figure 2. Venn diagram of the active compounds tested in propidium iodide, lactate quantification, and WormAssay. The diagram represents the distribution of the active compounds according to stage and used methods. The schistosomula assay using staining with PI is identified by the color green, schistosomula assay using the quantitative analysis of lactate is identified by the color yellow, the test in male adult worms by WormAssay is indicated by the color blue, and the test in female adult worms by WormAssay is represented by the color red.

Our work demonstrates the need to use parallel and complementary methods, since only using PI, for example, a lower number of compounds would be selected as active and consequently, potential compounds would be excluded. In view of the foregoing methods, the contributions from studies aimed at identifying new therapeutic compounds against schistosomiasis could, perhaps, be most effective if they employ more than a single method for screening drugs and different parasite stages. The association of fluorescence with PI staining enables the selection of compounds capable of altering parasite viability and/or inducing mortality. Moreover, male and female adult worms develop and have different metabolisms, and thus, their susceptibility to a specific drug also differs. One clear example is the studies demonstrating that female adult worms are more sensitive to praziquantel than males [4, 42] and approximately 1341 genes are up-regulated in female adult worms when compared to male [43]. Regarding the different life stages, results demonstrate that some drugs, including praziquantel, are active solely in the mature stage of *S. mansoni* [44].

These results indicate the need to employ different methods for drug screening as one can find a larger number of hits than when the tests are performed using only one method or in only one stage of the parasite. In addition, it substantiates the importance of using the selective approach to find active compounds, thus using a rational approach targeting previous validated targets, allowing direct design of specific compounds.

5. Validation of *S. mansoni* drug targets

The most common strategies used in drug discovery are the empirical and the rational approaches. The first is based on testing various compounds randomly looking for biological activities. The second is also called the selective approach as it proposes identifying a biological target and then designing or looking for a specific inhibitor for that target. In this sense, there are many strategies to assess gene function in parasites in order to elucidate their role in development, mechanisms of drug resistance, and speculate its use as a parasite control method. Among them, we can mention comparative "omics," RNA interference, heterologous complementation using model organisms (i.e., *Caenorhabditis elegans*) and *in silico* approaches. Comparative "omics" has been used to identify potential target proteins that appear to be essential for the parasite, while RNA interference has been used to validate a variety of drug target molecules, such as histone-modifying enzymes (HMEs), protein kinases, and others.

5.1. Histone-modifying enzymes

Among the most studied targets are epigenetic modulators, and among them are regulators of chromatin epigenetic modifications, named histone-modifying enzymes (HMEs), which act on the epigenome resulting in a change in the gene transcription profile. HMEs are involved in a wide range of reactions including methylation, demethylation, acetylation, deacetylation, phosphorylation, ADP-ribosylation, deimination, sumoylation, ubiquitination, etc. Yet, recent findings have described a myriad of lysine modifications, among others: formylation, succinylation, crotonylation, and malonylation [45].

The enzymes involved in the insertion and removal of methyl groups are called histone methyltransferase (HMT) and histone demethylases (HDM) [46]. The histone-modifying enzymes involved in the insertion and removal of acetyl groups are called histone acetyltransferases (HAT) and histone deacetylases (HDAC and sirtuins). Acetylation of lysine residues and methylation of lysine and/or arginine residues in histones H3 and H4 tails are two changes of particular importance [47, 48]. The insertion of acetyl and methyl groups neutralizes the positive charge of histones, destabilizing the structure of nucleosome and allowing the DNA to separate from histones, This results in the facilitation of the access of transcription factors and RNA polymerase to the DNA stimulating gene expression. The removal of these groups has the opposite effect, increasing the positive charge, condensing chromatin, and thereby, repressing transcription [49]. The heterochromatin is transcriptionally inactive when highly methylated at lysine 9 of histone H3 and not methylated at lysine 4, and hypoacetylated in histones H3 and H4 [50]. It is important to highlight that HDACs and sirtuins also deacetylate other nonhistone substrates such as chaperones, peroxiredoxins, transcription factors, signaling mediators, and structural proteins (e.g., [51–55]).

These modifications allow specific combinations that affect the overall structure of chromatin and the transcription of genes, the so-called histone code, which is, in many cases, conserved among organisms [50]. Aberrant epigenetic states are often associated with human diseases such as cancer, inflammation, metabolic, and neuropsychiatric disorders, and thus HMEs are implicated and intensively studied as therapeutic targets in various diseases [56–59].

One of the most promising approaches for drug discovery among HMEs is the development of HDAC inhibitors, which targets the highly studied lysine deacetylases. These targets are also key for parasites, including schistosomes, which present, similarly to tumors, dependence on lactate fermentation as energy source, host independent growth, high metabolic activity, and host immune evasion through mimetism of molecules [60]. In addition to schistosomes, HMEs have been highly explored as drug targets for parasitic diseases such as *Trypanosoma brucei*, *Plasmodium falciparum*, *Leishmania* spp., *Toxoplasma* sp., among others [61–63].

Many different types of HDAC inhibitors (HDACi) are under development. The inhibitors targeting class I and II HDACs are classified into four families according to their structure: inhibitors containing short-chain fatty acids (butyrate and the valproic acid—VPA), compounds derived from hydroxamic acid (the Trichostatin A—TSA and the acid-suberoylanilide hydroxamic—SAHA or vorinostat), and the group of cyclic tetrapeptides and benzamides. Among these inhibitors, SAHA was approved by Food and Drug Administration (FDA) for use in adult individuals with cutaneous T-cell lymphoma [64]. *In vitro* tests with butyrate, VPA and TSA, performed with human cells demonstrated that these inhibitors lead to apoptosis, differentiation, and cell cycle arrest [65].

Some studies have shown that HDACi, such as TSA, triggers histone H4 hyperacetylation in *S. mansoni* schistosomula at low concentration (2 µM), leading to apoptosis and affecting significantly gene transcription [66, 67]. According to Pierce and collaborators [65], *in vitro* exposure of schistosomula and adult worms with VPA inhibitors (TSA and SAHA) inhibited 80% of the total HDAC activity and caused the death of parasites.

In addition to pan HDAC inhibitors, one international consortium has been focusing in strategic epigenetic druggable targets for diverse parasites [65]. Recently, SmHDAC8 has risen as a promising target to treat schistosomiasis. First, SmHDAC8 was validated and proved to be essential for parasite infectivity, since parasites knocked down for SmHDAC8 were unable to normally develop in the mammalian host and showed, approximately, 50% reduction in oviposition [68]. Structural analysis has also shown that HDAC8 of *S. mansoni* presents important structural differences when compared to the human orthologue, despite a single amino acid substitution in the active site [68]. In this work, schistosomula larvae were exposed to hydroxamate derivative, HDAC8-specific inhibitor (J1075), which led to apoptosis and parasite death. These studies are a proof of concept that HMEs are important therapeutic targets, and potential new drugs based on HDACi can be developed against schistosomiasis.

To date, a way to expand the repertoire of specific Schistosoma, HDACi is utilizing a "piggy-back" strategy, which accelerates the exploration for novel antischistosomal compounds. These strategies are founded in the principle of using structure-based inhibitors, previously validated for other illnesses or other targets, to add a variety of chemical scaffolds and backbones, facilitating the development of selective inhibitors specifically aiming the schistosoma HMEs [69].

Besides deacetylases, HAT inhibitors and some derivatives of medicinal herbs, such as curcumin, also demonstrated their potential as inhibitors, since they induce hypoacetylation and lead tumor cells into apoptosis [70, 71]. Magalhães and collaborators [72] demonstrated the efficacy of curcumin in *S. mansoni*. In this study, the authors reported that in the presence of curcumin (5 and 20 µM), adult worms lose 50% of viability and reduce oviposition, and higher concentrations (50 and 100 µM) cause 100% mortality of worms. These data corroborate the results observed by our group, that 20 µM of this KDM1 and HAT inhibitor, causes a 95.5% motility reduction of female adult worms, confirming the importance of LSD1 and HAT for the development of *S. mansoni* (unpublished data).

Recent studies in *S. mansoni* demonstrated that the HAT inhibitor, PU139, at a high concentration (50 µM), affects adult worm pairing, the reproductive system of female adult worms, and the maturation of viable eggs [73]. In our hands, with a lower dose (20 µM), this compound was able to reduce female motility, confirming that it is active in the worm and highlighting the aforementioned (Section 2) necessity of assaying drug tests in female and male separately in order to reduce false negatives in drug screening in schistosomes.

Studies using HMT and HDM inhibitors are less common, but some results have shown that the chloroacetyl derivative, allantodapsone, a PRMT1 (arginine methyltransferase) inhibitor, showed selective inhibition affecting the growth of tumor cells [74]. Inhibitors of KDM1 (LSD1), a histone demethylase, are considered promising compounds for cancer therapy [75]. Studies performed by our group, knocked down for PRMT3 and KDMs in schistosomula by RNA interference, show that these enzymes are important for *S. mansoni* reproduction (unpublished data).

Due to the wide range of HME functions as "erasers" and "writers" of the epigenome, boosted by the use of histone and many nonhistone protein substrates, and taking into account the cellular localizations of these enzymes, it has been demonstrated, as expected, that they are essential and attractive targets for development of therapy for a number of infectious diseases, including schistosomiasis.

5.2. Protein kinases

The *Schistosoma* complex life cycle involves different life stages and requires sophisticated coordination of its physiological systems to ensure success of infection and survival in both hosts. Therefore, signals of the environment and hosts stimulate physiological, morphological, and biochemical changes [76, 77]. It involves nonlinear signaling networks that switch protein activity by phosphorylation (by protein kinases—PKs) and dephosphorylation (by protein phosphatases) of amino acid residues, or by incorporation of GTP. Protein kinase phosphorylation and the subsequent activation of signaling cascades result in the activation of transcription factors that target specific genes promoting or blocking their transcription. Furthermore, they can alter enzymatic activity, interaction with other proteins and molecules, cellular localization, and susceptibility to proteases degradation [78].

Eukaryotic protein kinases (ePKs) participate in phosphorylation cascades that regulate diverse cellular processes. PKs are among the largest gene families in eukaryotes and have been extensively studied and considered potential targets for drug development. The development of PK inhibitors has culminated in the approval of some drugs for the treatment of various human diseases such as cancer and diabetes. Furthermore, PKs have gained interest as potential drug targets against many parasites, including *S. mansoni* [79–82].

The *S. mansoni* predicted proteome is composed of about 2% of PKs, a total of 252 proteins, of which only about 30 have some functional experimental evidence [83]. The scarcity of data on *S. mansoni* PKs has motivated studies that will contribute to a better understanding of the roles of this protein family in parasite development and survival.

Four mitogen-activated protein kinases (MAPKs) were studied by our group using double-stranded RNA-mediated interference to elucidate their functional roles. Mice were infected with schistosomula after gene knockdown, and the development of adult worms was observed. Andrade et al. [79] showed that c-Jun N-terminal kinase SmJNK participates in the maturation and survival of the parasite, associated with the presence of undifferentiated oocytes and damage in the adult male tegument. SmERK-1 and SmERK-2 are involved in egg production, since females were recovered with undeveloped ovaries and immature oocytes, and the infected mice harbored significantly fewer eggs. Furthermore, the Smp38 kinase seems to have an important role in the development and survival of parasites and in their protection against reactive oxygen species (unpublished data). Thus, we demonstrated that MAPK proteins are important for parasite survival *in vivo* and are essential for the development and reproduction of the parasite.

Guidi et al. [84] used RNA interference to investigate the function of 24 proteins in adult worms and schistosomula, and among those, kinases were included. For atypical protein kinase C (SmaPKC), knockdown resulted in decreased viability in both stages. Knockdown of polo-like kinase 1 (SmPLK1) and p38 MAPK (Smp38) increased mortality only in larvae. The SmPLK1 inhibition with BI2536, a specific inhibitor, also increased mortality and interfered with egg production. Knockdown of SmPLK1 and SmaPKC also resulted in lower worm recoveries *in vivo*.

Ressurreição et al. [85] reported that phosphorylation of PKC, ERK, and p38 MAPK kinases is modulated by light and temperature. Furthermore, in response to linoleic acid, these kinases appear to coordinate the release of components of the cercarial acetabular gland, and PKC and ERK, when activated, are located in putative sensory receptors in the tail, thus demonstrating the importance of PKC, ERK, and p38 MAPK signaling pathways in the mechanisms for host penetration.

As mentioned, PKs are conserved and widely studied in many organisms; therefore, a range of PK inhibitors is already available, which are valuable tools. The function of some kinases was studied by parasite exposure to these inhibitors to explore PK functions in *S. mansoni*. Matsuyama et al. [86] demonstrated that cAMP-dependent protein kinase is involved in the osmosis-regulated ciliary movement of miracidia by exposure to the inhibitors PKI(14-22)amide, H89, and H88, verifying the complete inhibition of miracidia swimming in artificial pond water. Inhibition of protein kinase C (SmPKC) by GF109203X accelerates the rate of larval development of *S. mansoni*, with miracidia shedding its ciliary plates significantly faster and developing into mother sporocyst [87]. Another example, the polo-like kinase SmPlk1 has a potent and selective inhibitor (the anticancer drug BI 2536), which induces changes in schistosome gonads, an indication that SmPlk1 participates in parasite gametogenesis [88]. More recently, Long et al. [89] showed that knockdown of SmPlk1 using RNA interference induced abnormal phenotypes in schistosomula. They also tested a panel of 38 benzimidazole thiophene PLK1 inhibitors and 11 commercially available human PLK1 inhibitors in schistosomula and adult worms using microscopical observation and the QDREC approaches to verify changes in the parasite. Many of these inhibitors caused deleterious changes in the parasite.

Knobloch et al. [90] used the inhibitor Herbimycin A to demonstrate that protein tyrosine kinases (PTKs) regulates gonad development and egg production through changes in gene expression of eggshell proteins, and suggested PTKs as novel anti-*Schistosoma* drug targets. Transcriptome analyses of female worms after treatment with the inhibitors Herbimycin A and TRIKI, or both, revealed a number of genes that were transcriptionally affected. Herbimycin A specifically inhibited the Src kinase SmTK3, and TRIKI (TGF-β receptor type I kinase inhibitor) inhibited the TGFβ receptor, SmTβR. The expression of genes with recognized function in eggshell formation was investigated using quantitative polymerase chain reaction (qPCR) and proved to be regulated by the signaling pathways containing Src and TβRI [91].

Imatinib, an Abl-kinase-specific inhibitor used in human cancer therapy, was tested against adult worms and caused effects on morphology and physiology of *S. mansoni* couples *in vitro* [92]. Transcriptome analyses of adult worms treated with imatinib were performed using microarray and qPCR. Genes related to surface, muscle, gut, and gonad processes were differentially expressed. In addition, a comparative analysis of microarray data with previous data after TRIKI inhibition was performed and provided evidence of an association between TGFβ and Abl kinase signaling pathways [93].

Syk kinase (SmTK4) function was studied in adult worms using RNA interference and the specific inhibitor piceatannol. Prominent morphological changes in testes and ovaries were observed, demonstrating the role of SmTK4 in gametogenesis. In addition, the authors used yeast two-/three-hybrid library screenings and identified a Src kinase (SmTK6) acting upstream and a MAPK-activating protein and a mapmodulin acting downstream of SmTK4 [94].

A set of commercial kinase inhibitors was tested by Morel et al. [95] in schistosomula and adult worms, conforming deleterious effects on parasite physiology, as well as the importance of kinases in parasite biology and reproduction. In that study, five protein kinase B (SmPKB or SmAkt) inhibitors were tested and three affected pairing and oviposition of adult worms, in addition cause mortality in larvae. These data, along with other studies [96], suggest that SmAkt is a key regulator of schistosoma reproduction processes [95].

The roles of protein kinases C (PKCs) and extracellular signal-regulated kinases (ERKs) were studied through modulation of PKC and ERK activity by kinase activators and inhibitors in adult worms. Results have shown that this modulation induced worm uncoupling, suppressed egg output, male worm detachment, worm paralysis, and provoked sustained coiling. The authors also reported that praziquantel, the drug of choice for schistosomiasis treatment, induced activation of *S. mansoni* PKCs and ERKs. Activated PKC and ERK in adult worms are associated with muscular, tegumental, and reproductive structures [97].

5.3. Other targets

In addition to epigenetic modification, effectors and protein kinases, numerous proteins related to proteolytic, xenobiotic metabolism, redox processes, nucleotide biosynthesis and proteins involved in the nervous system of *Schistosoma* have been tested as therapeutic targets.

5.3.1. Peptidases

Peptidases are enzymes that perform proteolytic reactions and peptide bond hydrolysis. *Schistosoma mansoni* peptidases are attractive drug targets because they act in the host-parasite interaction during parasite invasion, migration, nutrition, and immune evasion [98]. The parasite serine peptidase involved in skin penetration of the human host, called cercarial elastase (SmCE), has been well studied [99, 100]. SmCE could have a role in immune evasion, as a highly purified SmCE was able to cleave IgE and other key molecules involved in immune regulation [101]. The use of serine protease inhibitors prevented IgE cleavage by cercariae and schistosomula extracts in a previous study, indicating that this could be a promising path for therapeutic strategies [102].

The *S. mansoni* cysteine and aspartic peptidases have drawn attention of many researchers as they participate in digestion of the blood meal. A previous study has shown that the use of inhibitors of these peptidases impairs hemoglobin degradation and arrests schistosome development and egg production [103]. The *S. mansoni* cathepsin B1 (SmCB1), which is a highly abundant digestive protease, was the focal point of various studies (reviewed in Ref. [104]). SmCB1 has been validated as a molecular target for therapy against schistosomiasis in a murine model of *S. mansoni* infection [105]. Moreover, SmCB1 crystal structure was determined, and specific inhibitors were designed, which are potential drug leads [106–108]. Another schistosome aspartic peptidase under study as a target is cathepsin D (SmCD). Morales et al. [109] have shown that silencing SmCD transcripts by RNA interference promoted schistosomula growth retardation as well as reduced worm and egg burden in infected mice. SmCD is currently under consideration for vaccine development against *S. mansoni* [110].

Prolyl oligopeptidases of the S9 family of serine peptidases have been investigated in *S. mansoni* by Fajtová et al. [111] who characterized the *S. mansoni* prolyl oligopeptidase (SmPOP) activity and showed that it is localized in the tegument and parenchyma of adult worms and schistosomula. Additionally, the authors designed specific inhibitors of SmPOP that were able to induce schistosoma death, suggesting that SmPOP could be a potential target for antischistosomal drug development.

5.3.2. Xenobiotic metabolism

The biotransformation of xenobiotics involves pathways that can be divided into three phases: (I) oxidation, reduction, or hydrolysis of xenobiotics; (II) conjugation of metabolites with endogenous compounds; and (III) excretion of modified molecules through membrane-bound transport proteins [112]. The xenobiotic metabolism can be a promising area for drug development since it implicates mechanisms that the parasite uses to eliminate drugs or toxic compounds; additionally, it plays vital roles in providing essential molecules for parasite survival. Among the *S. mansoni* biotransformation proteins, the phase I enzyme CYP450 has been studied by Ziniel et al. [113] who demonstrated that CYP450 RNA interference-mediated knockdown resulted in worm death. Additionally, imidazole antifungal CYP450 inhibitors had schistosomicidal activity against adult and larval worms, and blocked embryonic development in the egg.

The glutathione S-transferase (GST) family, from biotransformation pathway phase II, has been extensively studied in schistosomes. The knockdown of SmGST26 and SmGST28 in sporocysts by dsRNA exposure increased their susceptibility to exogenous oxidative stress and to *Biomphalaria glabrata* hemocytes-mediated killing [114]. The GST family of proteins is currently important vaccine candidate as it has been shown that these enzymes bind to several commercially available anthelmintics [115, 116].

The phase III membrane-bound transport proteins are currently under study, and the ABC transporters are the most studied among them [117]. The involvement of these ABC transporters such as P-glycoprotein and multidrug resistance-associated protein (SmDR1, SmDR2, SmMRP1, ABCA4, ABCB6, and ABCC10/MRP7) in drug susceptibility and development of drug resistance in schistosomes is clear, and this makes them excellent candidate targets for inhibitors that could potentiate the effect of existing drugs against schistosomes [118] or as new therapeutic targets themselves [119].

5.3.3. Redox mechanisms

Redox balance mechanisms are essential for schistosome worm survival, and differences between schistosome and human host redox networks were shown in previous studies (reviewed in Ref. [120]). The *S. mansoni* thioredoxin glutathione reductase (SmTGR) has been shown to be an important drug target. The use of oxadiazole-2-oxides as novel TGR inhibitors produced significant activity against various *S. mansoni* stages *ex vivo* and *in vivo* [40, 121, 122]. Another drug target in schistosome redox biology is the peroxiredoxins (SmPrx), which may be responsible to neutralize H_2O_2 due to the fact that schistosomes lack the catalase enzyme, resulting in a limited capacity to cope with this oxidant [120]. Sayed et al. [123] have shown that SmPrx1 knockdown by dsRNA exposure can potentially lead to schistosome death. *Schistosoma mansoni* antioxidant system relevance was also demonstrated in sporocysts by Mourão et al. [114]. RNAi-mediated knockdown of glutathione peroxidase (SmGPx), SmPrx1, and SmPrx2 increased larvae susceptibility to H_2O_2 oxidative stress. Additionally, treatment of parasites with SmPrx1/2 dsRNA increased hemocyte-mediated killing *in vitro*.

5.3.4. Purine biosynthesis

The purine nucleotide *de novo* synthesis pathway is absent in S. *mansoni*, which makes the parasite purine salvage pathway an attractive target for antischistosomal therapy development. A key component of this pathway is the purine nucleoside phosphorylase. The S. *mansoni* purine nucleoside phosphorylase (SmPNP) activity and structure have been well characterized [124–126]. Selective inhibitors for SmPNP have been tested in enzymatic assays *in vitro*; however, experiments with parasite larval or adult stages have not been reported yet [127–129]. The hypoxanthine-guanine phosphoribosyltransferase (HGPRTase) was also considered as a potential drug target [130]. Pereira et al. [131] performed with siRNA directed against SmHGPRTase the first successful demonstration of an *in vivo* RNAi-based treatment against schistosomiasis.

5.3.5. Neurotransmitter transporters

Schistosoma mansoni nervous system is very well developed with a rich diversity of neurotransmitters. The neurotransmitter serotonin is one of the most abundant neuroactive substances in the S. *mansoni* nervous system [132], stimulating worm movement, muscle contraction, glycogenolysis, and glucose utilization in schistosomes [133, 134]. The S. *mansoni* serotonin transporter (SmSERT) function and localization have been studied [135, 136], and apparently, it acts as a neuronal transporter playing a key role in serotonergic control of parasite motility. Some classical selective serotonin reuptake inhibitors that usually target this type of transporters have shown potent schistosomicidal effect in drug screening [10, 137]. Some of these inhibitors presented different potency and selectivity for SmSERT when compared to the human hSERT, indicating that this evolutionary distance could be explored for the development of novel anti-*Schistosoma* therapies.

The inhibitory neurotransmitters, norepinephrine (NE) and dopamine (DA), are also present in S. *mansoni*, and they cause muscular relaxation and worm body lengthening [134]. A dopamine/norepinephrine transporter (DAT) from S. *mansoni* (SmDAT) has been characterized [138], and it would be responsible for clearance of NE and DA following their release to terminate the signal. SmDAT pharmacological studies showed that its response to tricyclic antidepressants and to selective serotonin reuptake inhibitors was higher than that shown for human DAT. Once again, the differences in ligand binding activity of schistosome neurotransmitter transporters reinforce them as good candidates for selective drug targeting. Nevertheless, inhibitors of schistosome neurotransmitter transporters have not been tested in an animal infection model yet, so the concerns over psychoactivity and undesirable side effects in the host could not be ruled out.

5.3.6. Neurotransmitter receptors

The S. *mansoni* genome sequence predicts several putative neurotransmitter receptors from the two main classes: ligand-gated ion channels and G protein-coupled receptors (GPCR) [139]. Receptors of neurotransmitters dopamine, histamine, glutamate, serotonin, and acetylcholine have been cloned and characterized [140–147]. Many of these receptors have shown divergences from host receptors in structural and pharmacological aspects, indicating a possible track for antischistosomal therapy development. MacDonald et al. [148] demonstrated through RNA interference phenotypic assay that the knockdown of *S. mansoni* GPCR for acetylcholine (SmGAR) can disrupt larval motility. The importance of a serotonin receptor (Sm5HTR) for parasite motor activity has been also demonstrated by RNA interference [145]. Furthermore, it has been shown that the use of a heterologous system based on a fluorescent mammalian cell high-throughput functional assay can contribute as a new tool in the search for schistosomicidal drugs in the neurotransmitter receptors field [144].

6. Future directions and new approaches

While schistosomiasis still has a high socioeconomic impact, with the total number of disability-adjusted life years (DALY) lost to schistosomiasis estimated at 4.5 million per year, and treatment relies only on praziquantel since the early 1980s, drug discovery is still of great relevance. Our results with a *S. mansoni* drug screening platform reinforce that the use of parallel and complementary methods to assess parasites viability is essential in future studies. Drug discovery studies that employ different methods for drug screening are more prone to find new lead compounds. Additionally, drug screening should be performed in more than one parasite stages as some compound may present activity in schistosomula larval stage but be inactive in the adult worm stage or vice versa. It is worth to mention that praziquantel has little effect on immature worms; however, this drug acts in <1 h on adult worms damaging the tegument and paralyzing the worms. A compound that acts in all parasite stages and in both sexes is desirable, as such drug could be used to combat the acute and chronic phases of schistosomiasis, as well as to prevent the dissemination of viable eggs.

It is noteworthy that after identifying potential anti-*Schistosoma mansoni* drugs, several strict tests for validation are needed, those include bioavailability, stability, absorption, metabolism, distribution, excretion/pharmacokinetics, and toxicity in *in vivo* assays. The present chapter depicted the most studied drug targets on *S. mansoni*. The extensive publications on *Schistosoma* gene characterization studies and selective inhibitors design may pave the way for new therapeutic approaches against schistosomiasis.

Acknowledgements

This work has been supported by funding from the European Commission's Seventh Framework Programme for research, under Grant agreement no. 602080 (A-ParaDDisE), CAPES Programa PCDD-Programa CAPES/Nottingham University (3661/2014), FAPEMIG (CBB-APQ-00520-13). GO received funds from CNPq (470673/2014-1 and 309312/2012-4) and is funded by CAPES (003/2014, REDE 21/2015), CNPq (304138/2014-2), and FAPEMIG (PPM-00189-13).

Author details

Naiara Clemente Tavares[1], Pedro Henrique Nascimento de Aguiar[1], Sandra Grossi Gava[1], Guilherme Oliveira[2] and Marina Moraes Mourão[1*]

*Address all correspondence to: marinamm@cpqrr.fiocruz.br

1 Rene Rachou Research Center, FIOCRUZ, Belo Horizonte, Minas Gerais, Brazil

2 Vale Institute of Technology – ITV, Belém, Pará, Brazil

References

[1] Hotez PJ, Fenwick A. Schistosomiasis in Africa: an emerging tragedy in our new global health decade. PLoS Negl Trop Dis 2009; 3: e485.

[2] Gryseels B. Schistosomiasis. Infect Dis Clin North Am 2012; 26: 383–97.

[3] Botros S, Bennett J. Praziquantel resistance. Expert Opin Drug Discov 2007; 2: S35–S40.

[4] Coeli R, Baba EH, Araujo N, et al. Praziquantel treatment decreases Schistosoma mansoni genetic diversity in experimental infections. PLoS Negl Trop Dis 2013; 7: e2596.

[5] Liang YS, Dai J-RR, Zhu Y-CC, et al. Genetic analysis of praziquantel resistance in Schistosoma mansoni. Southeast Asian J Trop Med Public Health 2003; 34: 274–80.

[6] Melman SD, Steinauer ML, Cunningham C, et al. Reduced susceptibility to praziquantel among naturally occurring Kenyan isolates of Schistosoma mansoni. PLoS Negl Trop Dis 2009; 3: e504.

[7] Pica-Mattoccia L, Cioli D. Sex- and stage-related sensitivity of Schistosoma mansoni to in vivo and in vitro praziquantel treatment. Int J Parasitol 2004; 34: 527–33.

[8] Carvalho O dos S, Coelho PMZ, Lenzi HL. Schistosoma mansoni e esquistossomose: uma visão multidisciplinar. Rio de Janeiro: Editora Fiocruz, 2008.

[9] Suggitt M, Bibby MC. 50 Years of preclinical anticancer drug screening: Empirical to target-driven approaches. Clin Cancer Res 2005; 11: 971–981.

[10] Abdulla M-H, Ruelas DS, Wolff B, et al. Drug discovery for schistosomiasis: hit and lead compounds identified in a library of known drugs by medium-throughput phenotypic screening. PLoS Negl Trop Dis 2009; 3: e478.

[11] Rinaldi G, Loukas A, Brindley PJ, et al. Viability of developmental stages of Schistosoma mansoni quantified with xCELLigence worm real-time motility assay (xWORM). Int J Parasitol Drugs Drug Resist 2015; 5: 141–148.

[12] Keiser J. In vitro and in vivo trematode models for chemotherapeutic studies. Parasitology 2010; 137: 589–603.

[13] Inglese J, Johnson RL, Simeonov A, et al. High-throughput screening assays for the identification of chemical probes. Nat Chem Biol 2007; 3: 466–79.

[14] Lee H, Moody-Davis A, Saha U, et al. Quantification and clustering of phenotypic screening data using time-series analysis for chemotherapy of schistosomiasis. BMC Genomics 2012; 13: S4.

[15] Soufan O, Ba-Alawi W, Afeef M, et al. Mining chemical activity status from high-throughput screening assays. PLoS One 2015; 10: 1–16.

[16] Lemieux GA, Liu J, Mayer N, et al. A whole-organism screen identifies new regulators of fat storage. Nat Chem Biol 2011; 7: 206–213.

[17] Howe S, Zöphel D, Subbaraman H, et al. Lactate as a novel quantitative measure of viability in Schistosoma mansoni drug sensitivity assays. Antimicrob Agents Chemother 2015; 59: 1193–1199.

[18] Marcellino C, Gut J, Lim KC, et al. WormAssay: a novel computer application for whole-plate motion-based screening of macroscopic parasites. PLoS Negl Trop Dis 2012; 6: e1494.

[19] Paveley RA, Mansour NR, Hallyburton I, et al. Whole organism high-content screening by label-free, image-based bayesian classification for parasitic diseases. PLoS Negl Trop Dis 2012; 6: 1–11.

[20] Smout MJ, Kotze AC, McCarthy JS, et al. A novel high throughput assay for anthelmintic drug screening and resistance diagnosis by real-time monitoring of parasite motility. PLoS Negl Trop Dis 2010; 4: e885.

[21] Tritten L, Silbereisen A, Keiser J. Nitazoxanide: In vitro and in vivo drug effects against Trichuris muris and Ancylostoma ceylanicum, alone or in combination. Int J Parasitol Drugs Drug Resist 2012; 2: 98–105.

[22] Mansour NR, Bickle QD. Comparison of microscopy and Alamar blue reduction in a larval based assay for schistosome drug screening. PLoS Negl Trop Dis 2010; 4: e795.

[23] Peak E, Chalmers IW, Hoffmann KF. Development and validation of a quantitative, high-throughput, fluorescent-based bioassay to detect schistosoma viability. PLoS Negl Trop Dis 2010; 4: e759.

[24] Krautz-Peterson G, Simoes M, Faghiri Z, et al. Suppressing glucose transporter gene expression in schistosomes impairs parasite feeding and decreases survival in the mammalian host. PLoS Pathog 2010; 6: e1000932.

[25] Faghiri Z, Camargo SMR, Huggel K, et al. The tegument of the human parasitic worm Schistosoma mansoni as an excretory organ: the surface aquaporin SmAQP is a lactate transporter. PLoS One 2010; 5: e10451.

[26] Massie CE, Lynch A, Ramos-Montoya A, et al. The androgen receptor fuels prostate cancer by regulating central metabolism and biosynthesis. EMBO J 2011; 30: 2719–33.

[27] Matos P, Horn JA, Beards F, et al. A role for the mitochondrial-associated protein p32 in regulation of trophoblast proliferation. Mol Hum Reprod 2014; 20: 745–755.

[28] de Moraes Mourão M, Dinguirard N, Franco GR, et al. Phenotypic screen of early-developing larvae of the blood fluke, schistosoma mansoni, using RNA interference. PLoS Negl Trop Dis 2009; 3: e502.

[29] Bowling T, Mercer L, Don R, et al. Application of a resazurin-based high-throughput screening assay for the identification and progression of new treatments for human african trypanosomiasis. Int J Parasitol Drugs Drug Resist 2012; 2: 262–270.

[30] Shimony O, Jaffe CL. Rapid fluorescent assay for screening drugs on Leishmania amastigotes. J Microbiol Methods 2008; 75: 196–200.

[31] Kotze AC, Clifford S, O'Grady J, et al. An in vitro larval motility assay to determine anthelmintic sensitivity for human hookworm and Strongyloides species. Am J Trop Med Hyg 2004; 71: 608–616.

[32] Storey B, Marcellino C, Miller M, et al. Utilization of computer processed high definition video imaging for measuring motility of microscopic nematode stages on a quantitative scale: 'The Worminator'. Int J Parasitol Drugs drug Resist 2014; 4: 233–43.

[33] Asarnow D, Rojo-Arreola L, Suzuki BM, et al. The QDREC web server: determining dose-response characteristics of complex macroparasites in phenotypic drug screens. Bioinformatics 2015; 31: 1515–8.

[34] Farah IO, Kariuki TM, King CL, et al. An overview of animal models in experimental schistosomiasis and refinements in the use of non-human primates. Lab Anim 2001; 35: 205–12.

[35] Pellegrino J, Katz N. Experimental chemotherapy of Schistosomiasis mansoni. Adv Parasitol 1968; 6: 233–90.

[36] Katz N, Couto FFB, Araújo N. Imatinib activity on Schistosoma mansoni. Mem Inst Oswaldo Cruz 2013; 108: 850–3.

[37] Pereira AC, Silva MLA e, Souza JM, et al. In vitro and in vivo anthelmintic activity of (-)-6,6'-dinitrohinokinin against schistosomula and juvenile and adult worms of Schistosoma mansoni. Acta Trop 2015; 149: 195–201.

[38] Araujo N, Mattos ACA de, Coelho PMZ, et al. Association of oxamniquine praziquantel and clonazepam in experimental Schistosomiasis mansoni. Mem Inst Oswaldo Cruz 2008; 103: 781–5.

[39] Lancelot J, Caby S, Dubois-Abdesselem F, et al. Schistosoma mansoni sirtuins: characterization and potential as chemotherapeutic targets. PLoS Negl Trop Dis 2013; 7: 1–13.

[40] Li T, Ziniel PD, He P, et al. High-throughput screening against thioredoxin glutathione reductase identifies novel inhibitors with potential therapeutic value for schistosomiasis. Infect Dis Poverty 2015; 4: 40.

[41] Yousif F, Wassel G, Boulos L, et al. Contribution to in vitro screening of Egyptian plants for schistosomicidal activity. Pharm Biol 2012; 50: 732–9.

[42] Mwangi IN, Sanchez MC, Mkoji GM, et al. Praziquantel sensitivity of Kenyan Schistosoma mansoni isolates and the generation of a laboratory strain with reduced susceptibility to the drug. Int J Parasitol Drugs Drug Resist 2014; 4: 296–300.

[43] Anderson L, Amaral MS, Beckedorff F, et al. Schistosoma mansoni egg, adult male and female comparative gene expression analysis and identification of novel genes by RNA-Seq. PLoS Negl Trop Dis 2015; 9: e0004334.

[44] Doenhoff MJ, Cioli D, Utzinger J. Praziquantel: mechanisms of action, resistance and new derivatives for schistosomiasis. Curr Opin Infect Dis 2008; 21: 659–67.

[45] Choudhary C, Weinert BT, Nishida Y, et al. The growing landscape of lysine acetylation links metabolism and cell signalling. Nat Rev Mol Cell Biol 2014; 15: 536–50.

[46] de la Cruz X, Lois S, Sánchez-Molina S, et al. Do protein motifs read the histone code? Bioessays 2005; 27: 164–75.

[47] Berger SL. Histone modifications in transcriptional regulation. Curr Opin Genet Dev 2002; 12: 142–148.

[48] Kouzarides T. Chromatin modifications and their function. Cell 2007; 128: 693–705.

[49] Cavalcante AGDM, de Bruin PFC. The role of oxidative stress in COPD: current concepts and perspectives. J Bras Pneumol 2009; 35: 1227–37.

[50] Jasencakova Z, Soppe WJJ, Meister A, et al. Histone modifications in Arabidopsis—high methylation of H3 lysine 9 is dispensable for constitutive heterochromatin. Plant J 2003; 33: 471–480.

[51] Dowling DP, Gantt SL, Gattis SG, et al. Structural studies of human histone deacetylase 8 and its site-specific variants complexed with substrate and inhibitors. Biochemistry 2008; 47: 13554–63.

[52] Haberland M, Montgomery RL, Olson EN. The many roles of histone deacetylases in development and physiology: implications for disease and therapy. Nat Rev Genet 2009; 10: 32–42.

[53] Beumer JH, Tawbi H. Role of histone deacetylases and their inhibitors in cancer biology and treatment. Curr Clin Pharmacol 2010; 5: 196–208.

[54] Delcuve GP, Khan DH, Davie JR. Roles of histone deacetylases in epigenetic regulation: emerging paradigms from studies with inhibitors. Clin Epigenet 2012; 4: 5.

[55] Van Dyke MW. Lysine deacetylase (KDAC) regulatory pathways: an alternative approach to selective modulation. ChemMedChem 2014; 9: 511–22.

[56] Falkenberg KJ, Johnstone RW. Histone deacetylases and their inhibitors in cancer, neurological diseases and immune disorders. Nat Rev Drug Discov 2014; 13: 673–91.

[57] Mottamal M, Zheng S, Huang T, et al. Histone deacetylase inhibitors in clinical studies as templates for new anticancer agents. Molecules 2015; 20: 3898–3941.

[58] Kumar R, Li D-Q, Müller S, et al. Epigenomic regulation of oncogenesis by chromatin remodeling. Oncogene 2016; 35: 4423–36.

[59] Wang Z, Xue X, Sun J, et al. An 'in-depth' description of the small non-coding RNA population of Schistosoma japonicum schistosomulum. PLoS Negl Trop Dis 2010; 4: e596.

[60] Oliveira G. Cancer and parasitic infections: similarities and opportunities for the development of new control tools. Rev Soc Bras Med Trop 2014; 47: 1–2.

[61] Ouaissi M, Ouaissi A. Histone deacetylase enzymes as potential drug targets in cancer and parasitic diseases. J Biomed Biotechnol 2006; 2006: 134–74.

[62] New M, Olzscha H, La Thangue NB. HDAC inhibitor-based therapies: Can we interpret the code? Mol Oncol 2012; 6: 637–656.

[63] Andrews KT, Haque A, Jones MK. HDAC inhibitors in parasitic diseases. Immunol Cell Biol 2012; 90: 66–77.

[64] Duvic M, Talpur R, Ni X, et al. Phase 2 trial of oral vorinostat (suberoylanilide hydroxamic acid, SAHA) for refractory cutaneous T-cell lymphoma (CTCL). Blood 2007; 109: 31–39.

[65] Pierce RJ, Dubois-Abdesselem F, Lancelot J, et al. Targeting schistosome histone modifying enzymes for drug development. Curr Pharm Des 2012; 18: 3567–78.

[66] Azzi A, Cosseau C, Grunau C. Schistosoma mansoni: developmental arrest of miracidia treated with histone deacetylase inhibitors. Exp Parasitol 2009; 121: 288–91.

[67] Dubois F, Caby S, Oger F, et al. Histone deacetylase inhibitors induce apoptosis, histone hyperacetylation and up-regulation of gene transcription in Schistosoma mansoni. Mol Biochem Parasitol 2009; 168: 7–15.

[68] Marek M, Kannan S, Hauser A-T, et al. Structural basis for the inhibition of histone deacetylase 8 (HDAC8), a key epigenetic player in the blood fluke Schistosoma mansoni. PLoS Pathog 2013; 9: e1003645.

[69] Marek M, Oliveira G, Pierce RJ, et al. Drugging the schistosome zinc-dependent HDACs: current progress and future perspectives. Future Med Chem 2015; 7: 783–800.

[70] Balasubramanyam K, Varier RA, Altaf M, et al. Curcumin, a novel p300/CREB-binding protein-specific inhibitor of acetyltransferase, represses the acetylation of histone/

nonhistone proteins and histone acetyltransferase-dependent chromatin transcription. J Biol Chem 2004; 279: 51163–71.

[71]   Stimson L, Rowlands MG, Newbatt YM, et al. Isothiazolones as inhibitors of PCAF and p300 histone acetyltransferase activity. Mol Cancer Ther 2005; 4: 1521–1532.

[72]   Magalhães LG, Machado CB, Morais ER, et al. In vitro schistosomicidal activity of curcumin against Schistosoma mansoni adult worms. Parasitol Res 2009; 104: 1197–1201.

[73]   Carneiro VC, de Abreu da Silva IC, Torres EJL, et al. Epigenetic changes modulate schistosome egg formation and are a novel target for reducing transmission of schistosomiasis. PLoS Pathog 2014; 10: e1004116.

[74]   Bissinger E-M, Heinke R, Spannhoff A, et al. Acyl derivatives of p-aminosulfonamides and dapsone as new inhibitors of the arginine methyltransferase hPRMT1. Bioorg Med Chem 2011; 19: 3717–31.

[75]   Wang J, Lu F, Ren Q, et al. Novel histone demethylase LSD1 inhibitors selectively target cancer cells with pluripotent stem cell properties. Cancer Res 2011; 71: 7238–7249.

[76]   Amiri P, Locksley RM, Parslow TG, et al. Tumour necrosis factor alpha restores granulomas and induces parasite egg-laying in schistosome-infected SCID mice. Nature 1992; 356: 604–7.

[77]   LoVerde PT, Hirai H, Merrick JM, et al. Schistosoma mansoni genome project: an update. Parasitol Int 2004; 53: 183–192.

[78]   Johnson GL, Lapadat R. Mitogen-activated protein kinase pathways mediated by ERK, JNK, and p38 protein kinases. Science 2002; 298: 1911–2.

[79]   Andrade LF De, Mourão MDM, Geraldo JA, et al. Regulation of Schistosoma mansoni development and reproduction by the mitogen-activated protein kinase signaling pathway. PLoS Negl Trop Dis 2014; 8: e2949.

[80]   Dissous C, Ahier A, Khayath N. Protein tyrosine kinases as new potential targets against human schistosomiasis. BioEssays 2007; 29: 1281–1288.

[81]   Naula C, Parsons M, Mottram JC. Protein kinases as drug targets in trypanosomes and Leishmania. Biochim Biophys Acta 2005; 1754: 151–159.

[82]   Ward P, Equinet L, Packer J, et al. Protein kinases of the human malaria parasite Plasmodium falciparum: the kinome of a divergent eukaryote. BMC Genomics 2004; 5: 79.

[83]   Andrade LF, Nahum LA, Avelar LGA, et al. Eukaryotic protein kinases (ePKs) of the helminth parasite Schistosoma mansoni. BMC Genomics 2011; 12: 215.

[84]   Guidi A, Mansour NR, Paveley R a, et al. Application of RNAi to genomic drug target validation in schistosomes. PLoS Negl Trop Dis 2015; 9: e0003801.

[85] Ressurreição M, Kirk RS, Rollinson D, et al. Sensory protein kinase signaling in Schistosoma mansoni cercariae: host location and invasion. J Infect Dis 2015; 212: 1787–97.

[86] Matsuyama H, Takahashi H, Watanabe K, et al. The involvement of cyclic adenosine monophosphate in the control of schistosome miracidium cilia. J Parasitol 2004; 90: 8–14.

[87] Ludtmann MHR, Rollinson D, Emery AM, et al. Protein kinase C signalling during miracidium to mother sporocyst development in the helminth parasite, Schistosoma mansoni. Int J Parasitol 2009; 39: 1223–1233.

[88] Dissous C, Grevelding CG, Long T. Schistosoma mansoni polo-like kinases and their function in control of mitosis and parasite reproduction. An Acad Bras Cienc 2011; 83: 627–635.

[89] Long T, Neitz RJ, Beasley R, et al. Structure-bioactivity relationship for benzimidazole thiophene inhibitors of polo-like kinase 1 (PLK1), a potential drug target in Schistosoma mansoni. PLoS Negl Trop Dis 2016; 10: e0004356.

[90] Knobloch J, Kunz W, Grevelding CG. Herbimycin A suppresses mitotic activity and egg production of female Schistosoma mansoni. Int J Parasitol 2006; 36: 1261–72.

[91] Buro C, Oliveira KC, Lu Z, et al. Transcriptome analyses of inhibitor-treated schistosome females provide evidence for cooperating Src-kinase and TGFß receptor pathways controlling mitosis and eggshell formation. PLoS Pathog 2013; 9: e1003448.

[92] Beckmann S, Grevelding CG. Imatinib has a fatal impact on morphology, pairing stability and survival of adult Schistosoma mansoni in vitro. Int J Parasitol 2010; 40: 521–526.

[93] Buro C, Beckmann S, Oliveira KC, et al. Imatinib treatment causes substantial transcriptional changes in adult Schistosoma mansoni in vitro exhibiting pleiotropic effects. PLoS Negl Trop Dis 2014; 8: e2923.

[94] Beckmann S, Buro C, Dissous C, et al. The Syk kinase SmTK4 of Schistosoma mansoni is involved in the regulation of spermatogenesis and oogenesis. PLoS Pathog 2010; 6: e1000769.

[95] Morel M, Vanderstraete M, Cailliau K, et al. Compound library screening identified Akt/PKB kinase pathway inhibitors as potential key molecules for the development of new chemotherapeutics against schistosomiasis. Int J Parasitol Drugs Drug Resist 2014; 4: 256–266.

[96] Vanderstraete M, Gouignard N, Cailliau K, et al. Venus kinase receptors control reproduction in the platyhelminth parasite Schistosoma mansoni. PLoS Pathog 2014; 10: e1004138.

[97]   Ressurreição M, De Saram P, Kirk RS, et al. Protein kinase C and extracellular signal-regulated kinase regulate movement, attachment, pairing and egg release in Schistosoma mansoni. PLoS Negl Trop Dis 2014; 8: e2924.

[98]   McKerrow JH, Caffrey C, Kelly B, et al. Proteases in parasitic diseases. Annu Rev Pathol Mech Dis 2006; 1: 497–536.

[99]   Ingram JR, Rafi SB, Eroy-Reveles AA, et al. Investigation of the proteolytic functions of an expanded cercarial elastase gene family in Schistosoma mansoni. PLoS Negl Trop Dis 2012; 6: e1589.

[100]   Yang Y, Wen YJ, Cai YN, et al. Serine proteases of parasitic helminths. Korean J Parasitol 2015; 53: 1–11.

[101]   Aslam A, Quinn P, McIntosh RS, et al. Proteases from Schistosoma mansoni cercariae cleave IgE at solvent exposed interdomain regions. Mol Immunol 2008; 45: 567–74.

[102]   Pleass RJ, Kusel JR, Woof JM. Cleavage of human IgE mediated by Schistosoma mansoni. Int Arch Allergy Immunol 2000; 121: 194–204.

[103]   Wasilewski MM, Lim KC, Phillips J, et al. Cysteine protease inhibitors block schistosome hemoglobin degradation in vitro and decrease worm burden and egg production in vivo. Mol Biochem Parasitol 1996; 81: 179–89.

[104]   Jílková A, Horn M, Řezáč P, et al. Activation route of the Schistosoma mansoni cathepsin B1 drug target: structural map with a glycosaminoglycan switch. Structure 2014; 22: 1786–98.

[105]   Abdulla M-H, Lim K-C, Sajid M, et al. Schistosomiasis mansoni: novel chemotherapy using a cysteine protease inhibitor. PLoS Med 2007; 4: e14.

[106]   Fanfrlík J, Brahmkshatriya PS, Řezáč J, et al. Quantum mechanics-based scoring rationalizes the irreversible inactivation of parasitic Schistosoma mansoni cysteine peptidase by vinyl sulfone inhibitors. J Phys Chem B 2013; 117: 14973–82.

[107]   Horn M, Jílková A, Vondrásek J, et al. Mapping the pro-peptide of the Schistosoma mansoni cathepsin B1 drug target: modulation of inhibition by heparin and design of mimetic inhibitors. ACS Chem Biol 2011; 6: 609–17.

[108]   Jílková A, Rezácová P, Lepsík M, et al. Structural basis for inhibition of cathepsin B drug target from the human blood fluke, Schistosoma mansoni. J Biol Chem 2011; 286: 35770í81.

[109]   Morales ME, Rinaldi G, Gobert GN, et al. RNA interference of Schistosoma mansoni cathepsin D, the apical enzyme of the hemoglobin proteolysis cascade. Mol Biochem Parasitol 2008; 157: 160–168.

[110]   Ahmad Fuaad AAH, Roubille R, Pearson MS, et al. The use of a conformational cathepsin D-derived epitope for vaccine development against Schistosoma mansoni. Bioorg Med Chem 2015; 23: 1307–12.

[111] Fajtová P, Štefanic S, Hradilek M, et al. Prolyl oligopeptidase from the blood fluke Schistosoma mansoni: from functional analysis to anti-schistosomal inhibitors. PLoS Negl Trop Dis 2015; 9: e0003827.

[112] Cvilink V, Lamka J, Skálová L. Xenobiotic metabolizing enzymes and metabolism of anthelminthics in helminths. Drug Metab Rev 2009; 41: 8–26.

[113] Ziniel PD, Karumudi B, Barnard AH, et al. The Schistosoma mansoni cytochrome P450 (CYP3050A1) is essential for worm survival and egg development. PLoS Negl Trop Dis 2015; 9: e0004279.

[114] Mourão MDM, Dinguirard N, Franco GR, et al. Role of the endogenous antioxidant system in the protection of Schistosoma mansoni primary sporocysts against exogenous oxidative stress. PLoS Negl Trop Dis 2009; 3: e550.

[115] Brophy PM, Barrett J. Glutathione transferase in helminths. Parasitology 1990; 100 Pt 2: 345–9.

[116] Mo AX, Agosti JM, Walson JL, et al. Schistosomiasis elimination strategies and potential role of a vaccine in achieving global health goals. Am J Trop Med Hyg 2014; 90: 54–60.

[117] Greenberg RM. Schistosome ABC multidrug transporters: from pharmacology to physiology. Int J Parasitol Drugs Drug Resist 2014; 4: 301–309.

[118] Kasinathan RS, Sharma LK, Cunningham C, et al. Inhibition or knockdown of ABC transporters enhances susceptibility of adult and juvenile schistosomes to praziquantel. PLoS Negl Trop Dis 2014; 8: 1–11.

[119] Kasinathan RS, Morgan WM, Greenberg RM. Genetic knockdown and pharmacological inhibition of parasite multidrug resistance transporters disrupts egg production in Schistosoma mansoni. PLoS Negl Trop Dis 2011; 5: e1425.

[120] Huang H-H, Rigouin C, Williams DL. The redox biology of schistosome parasites and applications for drug development. Curr Pharm Des 2012; 18: 3595–611.

[121] Sayed A a, Simeonov A, Thomas CJ, et al. Identification of oxadiazoles as new drug leads for the control of schistosomiasis. Nat Med 2008; 14: 407–412.

[122] Rai G, Sayed AA, Lea WA, et al. Structure mechanism insights and the role of nitric oxide donation guide the development of oxadiazole-2-oxides as therapeutic agents against schistosomiasis. J Med Chem 2009; 52: 6474–83.

[123] Sayed AA, Cook SK, Williams DL. Redox balance mechanisms in Schistosoma mansoni rely on peroxiredoxins and albumin and implicate peroxiredoxins as novel drug targets. J Biol Chem 2006; 281: 17001–17010.

[124] da Silveira NJF, Uchôa HB, Canduri F, et al. Structural bioinformatics study of PNP from Schistosoma mansoni. Biochem Biophys Res Commun 2004; 322: 100–4.

[125] Pereira HD, Franco GR, Cleasby A, et al. Structures for the potential drug target purine nucleoside phosphorylase from Schistosoma mansoni causal agent of schistosomiasis. J Mol Biol 2005; 353: 584–99.

[126] Pereira HM, Cleasby A, Pena S SDJ, et al. Cloning, expression and preliminary crystallographic studies of the potential drug target purine nucleoside phosphorylase from Schistosoma mansoni. Acta Crystallogr D Biol Crystallogr 2003; 59: 1096–9.

[127] Castilho MS, Postigo MP, Pereira HM, et al. Structural basis for selective inhibition of purine nucleoside phosphorylase from Schistosoma mansoni: kinetic and structural studies. Bioorg Med Chem 2010; 18: 1421–1427.

[128] De Moraes MC, Cardoso CL, Cass QB. Immobilized purine nucleoside phosphorylase from Schistosoma mansoni for specific inhibition studies. Anal Bioanal Chem 2013; 405: 4871–4878.

[129] Postigo MP, Guido RVC, Oliva G, et al. Discovery of new inhibitors of schistosoma mansoni PNP by pharmacophore-based virtual screening. J Chem Inf Model 2010; 50: 1693–1705.

[130] Craig SP, McKerrow JH, Newport GR, et al. Analysis of cDNA encoding the hypoxanthine-guanine phosphoribosyltransferase (HGPRTase) of Schistosoma mansoni; a putative target for chemotherapy. Nucleic Acids Res 1988; 16: 7087–101.

[131] Pereira TC, Pascoal VDB, Marchesini RB, et al. Schistosoma mansoni: evaluation of an RNAi-based treatment targeting HGPRTase gene. Exp Parasitol 2008; 118: 619–623.

[132] Bennett J, Bueding E, Timms AR, et al. Occurrence and levels of 5-hydroxytryptamine in Schistosoma mansoni. Mol Pharmacol 1969; 5: 542–5.

[133] Day TA, Bennett JL, Pax RA. Serotonin and its requirement for maintenance of contractility in muscle fibres isolated from Schistosoma mansoni. Parasitology 1994; 108 (Pt 4: 425–32.

[134] Pax RA, Siefker C, Bennett JL. Schistosoma mansoni: differences in acetylcholine, dopamine, and serotonin control of circular and longitudinal parasite muscles. Exp Parasitol 1984; 58: 314–24.

[135] Patocka N, Ribeiro P. Characterization of a serotonin transporter in the parasitic flatworm, Schistosoma mansoni: Cloning, expression and functional analysis. Mol Biochem Parasitol 2007; 154: 125–133.

[136] Patocka N, Ribeiro P. The functional role of a serotonin transporter in Schistosoma mansoni elucidated through immunolocalization and RNA interference (RNAi). Mol Biochem Parasitol 2013; 187: 32–42.

[137] Ribeiro P, Patocka N. Neurotransmitter transporters in schistosomes: structure, function and prospects for drug discovery. Parasitol Int 2013; 62: 629–638.

[138] Larsen MB, Fontana ACK, Magalhães LG, et al. A catecholamine transporter from the human parasite Schistosoma mansoni with low affinity for psychostimulants. Mol Biochem Parasitol 2011; 177: 35–41.

[139] Berriman M, Haas BJ, LoVerde PT, et al. The genome of the blood fluke Schistosoma mansoni. Nature 2009; 460: 352–8.

[140] El-Shehabi F, Ribeiro P. Histamine signalling in Schistosoma mansoni: immunolocalisation and characterisation of a new histamine-responsive receptor (SmGPR-2). Int J Parasitol 2010; 40: 1395–1406.

[141] El-Shehabi F, Vermeire JJ, Yoshino TP, et al. Developmental expression analysis and immunolocalization of a biogenic amine receptor in Schistosoma mansoni. Exp Parasitol 2009; 122: 17–27.

[142] El-Shehabi F, Taman A, Moali LS, et al. A novel G protein-coupled receptor of Schistosoma mansoni (SmGPR-3) is activated by dopamine and is widely expressed in the nervous system. PLoS Negl Trop Dis 2012; 6: e1523.

[143] Hamdan FF, Abramovitz M, Mousa A, et al. A novel Schistosoma mansoni G protein-coupled receptor is responsive to histamine. Mol Biochem Parasitol 2002; 119: 75–86.

[144] MacDonald K, Buxton S, Kimber MJ, et al. Functional characterization of a novel family of acetylcholine-gated chloride channels in Schistosoma mansoni. PLoS Pathog 2014; 10: e1004181.

[145] Patocka N, Sharma N, Rashid M, et al. Serotonin signaling in Schistosoma mansoni: a serotonin-activated G protein-coupled receptor controls parasite movement. PLoS Pathog 2014; 10: e1003878.

[146] Taman A, Ribeiro P. Investigation of a dopamine receptor in Schistosoma mansoni: functional studies and immunolocalization. Mol Biochem Parasitol 2009; 168: 24–33.

[147] Taman A, Ribeiro P. Glutamate-mediated signaling in Schistosoma mansoni: a novel glutamate receptor is expressed in neurons and the female reproductive tract. Mol Biochem Parasitol 2011; 176: 42–50.

[148] MacDonald K, Kimber MJ, Day TA, et al. A constitutively active G protein-coupled acetylcholine receptor regulates motility of larval Schistosoma mansoni. Mol Biochem Parasitol 2015; 202: 29–37.

6

Complex High-Content Phenotypic Screening

Shane R. Horman

Additional information is available at the end of the chapter

Abstract

There has been a renewed interest in cell-based phenotypic screening in drug discovery with the goal of improving the success and decreasing the clinical failure rate of new therapeutics. This has increasingly led to the development of biomimetic cellular models that more faithfully replicate human disease biology. Human tumour models have advanced to include relevant cell types such as primary patient tumour cells and grown using organotypic and 3D methods. Tissue organoids, which are 3D organ buds displaying realistic microanatomy, are becoming more commonly used in drug discovery to advance *in vitro* assays which predict drug toxicity and pharmacokinetics. Emerging technologies and cell culture methods are constantly improving the quality of tissue modelling that can be employed during primary phenotypic screening, and this has resulted in the identification of more efficacious and patient-relevant therapeutics.

Keywords: phenotypic, HTS, screening, high-content, high-throughput, three-dimensional, complex, spheroid, drug discovery, ECM, matrix

1. Introduction

This chapter will introduce the concept of complex and advanced high-content phenotypic drug screening. Phenotypic screening is a reductionist approach to modelling a particular aspect of biology and identifying modifiers of that biology. Conventionally, genomics- and chemical-based high-content screening has been performed on single cell types grown on plastic. However, accumulating evidence has shown that those methods are poor surrogates of actual disease biology. Three-dimensional and complex phenotypic screening employs disease-relevant cell types assembled in biomimetic fashion and miniaturized to accommodate a 384- or 1536-well high-content screening plate. Screening platforms for 3D and multi-culture cell models are typically employed in oncology research to better represent patient tumour biology. Recently, advanced cell culture techniques have made their way into other disease areas such as regenerative medicine and immunology, and the resulting screening platforms have greatly expanded the therapeutic targeting space.

2. What is phenotypic screening?

2.1. Description and historical significance of phenotypic screening

A phenotype is a composite of an organism's observable traits. On a cellular scale, a phenotype refers to a definable characteristic such as morphology, biochemical or physiological properties, motility or cell cycle status. A phenotypic assay is a quantitative measurement of one or more cellular parameters after exposure to a modifying agent or perturbagen such as small molecules, proteins or RNA-interfering reagents. Application of a phenotypic assay to large-scale endeavours where many test reagents are applied to the cellular model is referred to as phenotypic screening. Phenotypic screening is regularly employed in early stage drug discovery by both academic and pharmaceutical institutions where it is referred to as phenotypic drug discovery (PDD). Phenotypic screening is a system-based approach using a target-agnostic assay to monitor phenotypic changes *in vitro* or *in vivo* [1]. PDD is often carried out in a high-content or high-throughput fashion using microtiter plates with 96, 384 or 1536 wells (**Figure 1**) to enable the analysis of thousands or millions of test compounds.

Phenotypic screening is not a new concept. In fact, before the era of cellular biology phenotypic screening was often carried out in whole organisms. A benchmark example of this process was the large scale systematic screening to find a drug against syphilis. In 1909, the Nobel Prize-winning immunologist Ehrlich et al. synthesized hundreds of organoarsenic derivatives and tested them in syphilis-infected rabbits [2]. The 606th series tested cured the rabbits and was later marketed as Salvarsan, which was one of the most frequently prescribed drugs until its replacement by penicillin in the 1940s [3]. Alexander Fleming, arguably the most well-known microbiologist of recent history and discoverer of penicillin, pioneered the first type of *in vitro* antimicrobial screening technique. He would use small circles of filter paper doused in a test chemical and applied to a lawn of pathogenic bacteria in a Petri dish to look for zones of growth inhibition (**Figure 2**). This method, eventually optimized in the 1950s as the Kirby-Bauer disk diffusion test, required much less resources than testing in diseased animal models and eventually became an industry standard for the systematic identification of new antimicrobial compounds [3]. This technique is still widely used in academia and industry, though at a much higher throughput.

Modern phenotypic screening in eukaryotic cells arose with the capacity to culture human cells *in vitro*. Although mammalian cells have been propagated *in vitro* since 1907 [4], cell culture techniques advanced significantly in the 1940s and 1950s to support efforts in virology research. The basis for conventional cancer drug discovery began with the emergence of human cancer cell lines in the 1950s, starting with the well-known HeLa cell line [5]. Since that time, many human tumour cells from all types of solid organs and hematopoietic cancers have been adapted to *in vitro* cell culture conditions and used to find new drugs that kill cancer cells. Early phenotypic screening from the 1960s through the 1990s relied heavily on cytotoxic assays that identified anticancer drugs in human cell lines that exhibit the phenotype of rapid unrestrained growth [6]. Arguably the most successful examples from those efforts were the discoveries of camptothecin and taxol in the 1960s which are still widely used to treat many types of cancer. However, with the advent of modern genomics and its application to the study of cancer genomes, tumour transcriptional profiles and disease-driving mutations, a revised understanding of the molecular bases of cancer has yielded new classifications of tumour cell phenotypes [7]. This nuanced view of the molecular underpinnings of cancer has facilitated more rapid target-based drug discovery (TDD) but also enabled the definition of more patient-relevant cellular models and phenotypes that can be employed in PDD. Subsequently, modern phenotypic screening initiatives involve somewhat more knowledge of the disease biology and are not entirely target-agnostic compared to earlier "black box" screening efforts.

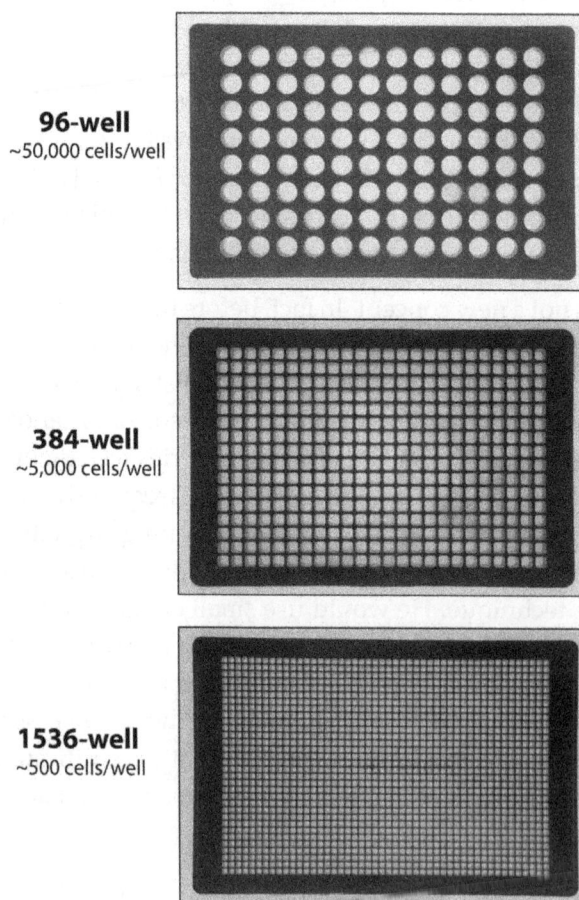

96-well
~50,000 cells/well

384-well
~5,000 cells/well

1536-well
~500 cells/well

Figure 1. Three different assay plate formats used in high-content cell culture. The 96-well plate is rarely used in drug discovery and is only for assays incapable of further miniaturization (screening capacity: 1000s of compounds). The 384-well plate is a standard size for complex phenotypic screening (screening capacity: 100,000s of compounds). The 1536-well plate is mainly used for biochemical and simple cell-based assays (screening capacity: 1,000,000s of compounds).

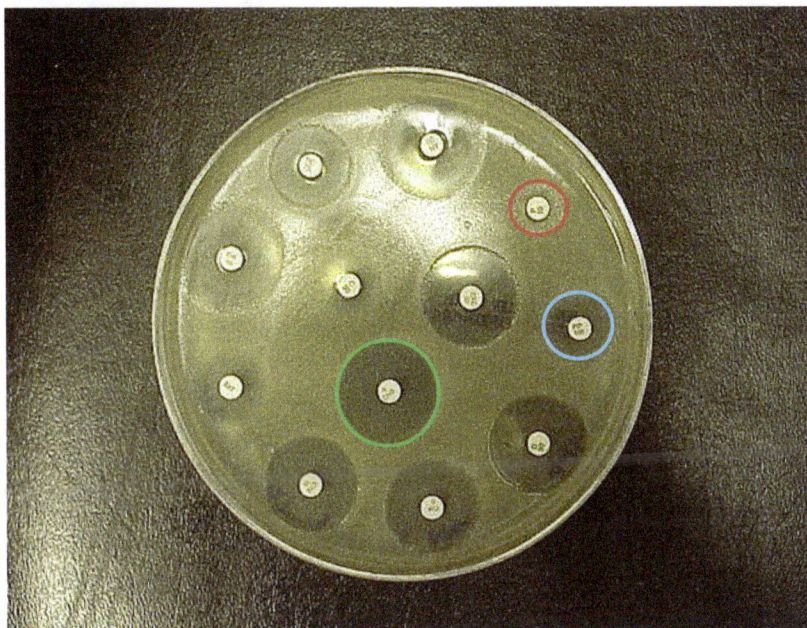

Figure 2. The Kirby-Bauer disk diffusion test. Pathogenic bacteria are plated as a lawn on a nutrient agar plate and paper disks containing test compounds are added. After 24–48 h, some disks display large zones of negative growth (green circle), moderate zones of negative growth (blue circle) or no effect (red circle). *Public image submitted by the U.S. National Oceanic and Atmospheric Administration.*

2.2. Phenotypic screening versus target-based screening

In terms of methods used to discover new drugs, phenotypic drug discovery is in stark contrast to target-based drug discovery (TDD), where the target (phenotype-modifying protein) is already known. Although target-based screening approaches may occur within cells, they often consist of biochemical assays using purified recombinant proteins in artificial environments. TDD is a rational, informed approach to drug discovery that uses molecular tools (compounds or biologics) to modify a particular target's activity or behaviour. Although TDD is the predominant form of drug discovery in big pharma, it relies on the unwavering assumption that the target in question is the elicitor of the relevant disease biology. Opposing this, a principle application of PDD is to identify new, previously unknown targets that may impact a phenotype hypothesized to be linked to disease pathology. Although TDD is a hypothesis-driven approach to identifying new drugs and also may provide criteria for choosing patient populations and setting doses, PDD has likely been more successful at identifying first-in-class medicines through the unbiased identification of novel molecular mechanisms of action (MMoA) [8].

The target-based approach (TDD) can be thought of as molecularly driven and involves the identification of chemical or biological reagents that modify the activity of one specific protein. Target-based drug discovery begins with a validated target protein that has been shown to convey an important aspect of the relevant disease biology. Therefore, in essence, the target-based approach is only as strong as the evidence produced for the characterization of that target. Perhaps, the most classic and well-defined example of target-based drug discovery is the discovery of Gleevec (imatinib) for the treatment of chronic myelogenous leukaemia (CML). In 1960, a chromosomal abnormality was discovered in the white blood cells of CML patients and dubbed the Philadelphia chromosome by the two researchers in Philadelphia who made the discovery [9]. However, it was not until 1973 that the Philadelphia (Ph) chromosome was characterized as a translocation between chromosomes 9 and 22 [10]. A further twelve years later, in 1985, the Ph chromosomal rearrangement was shown to yield the BCR-ABL fusion protein which was identified as the genetic driver of malignant neoplasia [11]. Finally, in 1993, a clinician in haematology/oncology named Brian Drucker teamed up with the Ciba-Geigy pharmaceutical company (now Novartis) to find a low molecular weight compound that could inhibit the BCR-ABL fusion protein and kill CML cells. The product of those efforts, a compound called STI571 and eventually known as imatinib, would go on to save thousands of lives and effectively cure Ph+ CML [12]. The Gleevec story is a textbook example of how target-based drug discovery is carried out in well-defined sequential steps: (1) a genetic abnormality in a diseased population is identified, (2) that genetic abnormality is shown to produce a mutant protein that drives the disease, and (3) a screening campaign identifies a chemical modulator of the mutant protein. Although the current field of molecular genomics now enables a faster turnaround time between the identification of a mutant protein and the chemical screen for a therapeutic, there still must exist a substantial body of work around the protein of interest to launch a full-blown drug discovery campaign.

Phenotypic drug discovery (PDD), on the other hand, is a discovery process that begins with an observable and quantifiable change in biology (phenotype) without prior knowledge of a causal target or mechanism of action. Due to the fact that modern phenotypic screening in drug discovery was only recently industrialized and the length of time needed to progress a drug from the bench to the bedside (10–15 years by most estimates), there are few examples of drugs currently being used in the clinic that were discovered from purely phenotypic-based approaches. Although taxol and camptothecin were discovered using cancer cell viability assays, a particularly inspiring example of PDD in recent history is the identification of vorinostat (Zolinza) for use in haematological malignancies. In 1971, an academic investigator at the Sloan-Kettering Institute for Cancer Research in New York made the observation that dimethyl sulfoxide (DMSO) had the properties of being able to induce erythroid differentiation in erythroleukaemia cells [13]. As leukaemia cells are often characterized by their lack of differentiated state, a compound capable of restoring differentiation in these cells is highly desirable. DMSO is an organosulfur fluid that is frequently used to dissolve both polar and non-polar compounds and is one of the most widely used reagents in chemistry and pharmaceutical discovery. The initial phenotypic observation led to the assembling and screening of DMSO-related and –derived compounds that had similar chemical structures. Although the set of compounds synthesized and screened in this effort would be considered small by today's comparison, the investigators were able to find one molecule, suberoylanilide hydroxamic acid (SAHA) that was able to induce cytodifferentiation and growth arrest of erythroleukaemia cells much more potently than DMSO. After many years of trial and error, SAHA was eventually moved to preclinical development after the discovery that its target was histone deacetylase (HDAC) [14]. RNA transcription and subsequent protein expression is regulated by acetylation of histone proteins, and HDACs have been shown to contribute to the development and progression of cancer through their silencing of tumour suppressor genes and/or activation of oncogenes. HDAC inhibitors and other epigenetic modifiers are now widely used in the clinic to treat a variety of hematopoietic malignancies and solid organ tumours. However, at the time of vorinostat preclinical development, HDAC inhibition was viewed as a completely novel approach to treating cancer. Several successful clinical trials showed that vorinostat was efficacious in treating patients with cutaneous T-cell lymphoma (CTCL), and the drug was approved by the FDA in 2006 [15]. Ensuing clinical trials showed that vorinostat is successful in treating other types of lymphoma, glioblastoma and non-small cell lung cancer and this has paved the way for other HDAC inhibitor development programs. Therefore, this drug, vorinostat, was derived from a common reagent present on the laboratory bench of nearly every pharmaceutical researcher and was shown by PDD to elicit a therapeutic mechanism completely novel to medicine.

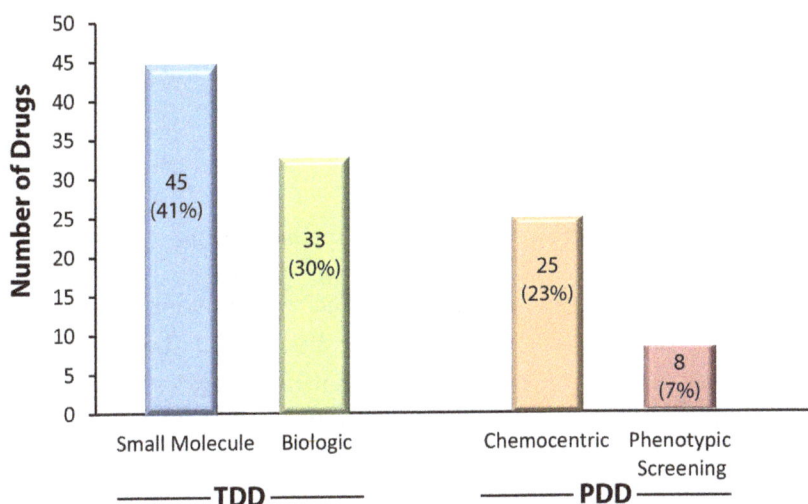

Figure 3. Discovery of first-in-class drugs approved by the US FDA from 1999 to 2013. Most drugs were discovered through target-based approaches (TDD) with more small molecule drugs (compounds) than biological ones (proteins). Most system-based approaches (e.g. PDD) originated from a known compound class (chemocentric) and relatively few were discovered by pure black box PDD. Adapted with permission from [1].

The true measure of which drug discovery approach is more successful, target-based or phenotypic-based, is how many drugs currently used in the clinic originated from each approach. Since the late 1990s, most pharmaceutical discovery has focused on target-based approaches, so there has been a heavy bias towards TDD compared to PDD. However, in terms of first-in-class drugs that target "new molecular entities" (NMEs), phenotypic approaches have been shown to be more successful than the target-based approaches that typically involve follower drugs or "me too drugs" [8]. Me too drugs are structurally similar to existing drugs and share the same target class, though they are distinct enough to escape patent infringement. Although these types of drugs may create competition between pharma companies and may drive drug prices down, within the research and development space, they may hamper creativity, innovation and ultimately, productivity. Conversely, a more recent review of the origins of 113 first-in-class drugs approved by the FDA from 1999 to 2013 revealed the majority (71%) of first-in-class drugs were discovered through target-based approaches (**Figure 3**) [1]. Regarding the systems-based approaches (e.g. PDD) for NMEs during this time frame, most drugs originated from a known compound or compound class (chemocentric approach) and only a few were discovered through purely target-agnostic phenotypic screening-based efforts (**Figure 3**) [1].

In the practical sense and from a pharma perspective, most drug discovery falls somewhere between TDD and PDD. Although a large portion of exploratory screening is performed in phenotypic models, the reagents that are screened are mechanistically informed. This has led to a newly defined approach that still falls under the category of phenotypic screening but is not entirely target-agnostic. Mechanism-informed phenotypic drug discovery (MIPDD) is screening against targets that are known or reported to be involved in the relevant disease pathology [6]. For example, screening ion channel inhibitors in cardiac assays or modifiers of extracellular matrix (ECM) remodelling for cartilage regeneration assays would be MIPDD. In essence, this approach restricts the scale of reagents tested but subsequently allows for easier data deconvolution due to the limited range of MoAs. This concept of MIPDD becomes especially important when designing and screening complex and 3D phenotypic cellular models, as will be discussed later.

2.3. Benefits and liabilities of high-content phenotypic screening

One problem in particular that plagues PDD but not TDD in high-content compound screening is target deconvolution. PDD is accompanied by the challenge of identifying what molecular entities are engaged by the hit compounds and what the phenotype-modifying molecular mechanism of action might be. Deconvoluting a compound's MMoA may not prove to be difficult assuming there are biomarkers or pharmacodynamic (PD) markers of compound action. For example, receptor internalization, reduced kinase phosphorylation or downregulated oncogene expression may explain a general MMoA, but it does not reveal the actual target of the compound. There are a variety of technologies available to identify the target(s) of a compound; for example, affinity chromatography, protein microarrays or chemical proteomics, though they each have their respective benefits and liabilities [16]. There are two main approaches to target deconvolution following phenotypic screening; the direct approach where the target is identified physically bound to the compound and the indirect approach that relies on cellular profiling. The direct approach method that provides the most confident data is chemical proteomics. Chemical proteomics involves the modification of one part of the compound so that it can be immobilized onto a purification bead (**Figure 4A** and **B**). The compound is then mixed with cellular extract and a pull-down assay followed by mass spectrometry reveals the most likely proteins that are bound to the modified compound (**Figure 4C**). Although this approach is the most straightforward, it is strictly dependent on knowing the active site(s) of the compound. The compound must be tethered to the bead in a manner that maintains its target recognition properties or the mass spec results may be misleading [16] (**Figure 4**).

From an early stage drug discovery perspective, it is more desirable to "fail early", than to progress a drug to later evaluation stages which are more time and resource consuming [18]. What this translates to is better selection of drug candidates early in the discovery process, possibly at the primary screening stage. One important reason invoked to play a role in the benefits of PDD over TDD is that PDD enables the testing of drug candidates in the context of the cell, and not in a biochemical assay using purified recombinant proteins as is typical with TDD. Since cell models are used in the prioritization of drug candidates based on potency and toxicity, it is only rational to bring those models forward to primary screening efforts to minimize late-stage expensive failures [19]. Therefore, it is critical that cell models of human disease used for primary high-content screens are as predictive of *in vivo* cellular biology as possible.

3. Paradigm shift in cell culture: 2D–3D

3.1. Recognizing the shortcomings of 2D cell models

If the purpose of drug discovery is the identification of novel chemical entities that alleviate a burden of infection or disease, then the diseased tissue in question should be accurately represented during the discovery process. What this translates to on the benchtop is a cellular model that is intended to faithfully replicate important aspects of disease as seen in a patient. Cells in the human body grow in 3D and are surrounded by other cells that continuously communicate to maintain organ function and homeostasis. Further, a variety of different extracellular matrices are found throughout the body that support cellular structure and organ integrity. The stimuli and responses experienced by cells *in vivo* is lost when those cells are purified and cultured in 2D on plastic or glass surfaces. Although 2D cell culture is relatively easy, robust and inexpensive, it may often misrepresent the biology of a phenotype. The key difference between 2D and 3D cell culture is cell-to-substrate interactions versus cell-to-cell interactions. Cells cultured on plastic assume a more flat and geometrically-constrained structure due to the interactions with the rigid substrate. This cell flattening can affect the spatial distribution of cell surface receptors and prevent the polarized morphology as seen *in vivo* [19]. Many important cell signalling pathways are downstream of cell surface receptors, and their misalignment can have serious and discrepant consequences. Integrins, for example, are cell surface receptors that communicate cell-to-cell and cell-to-ECM interactions and regulate the cytoskeleton. Integrins sense the extracellular microenvironment and activate protein signalling pathways inside the cell which results in proliferation, shape or motility changes and enables a rapid and flexible response to events occurring on the cell surface [20]. When cells are cultured on plastic, integrin expression and, subsequently, cellular behaviour can be drastically changed [20, 21]. These discrepancies can be further highlighted by comparing gene expression between the same cells grown as a 2D monolayer, 3D spheroid or subcutaneous tumour implant in a mouse (**Figure 6**). Comparative RNAseq studies highlight the massive batteries of genes that are turned off during 2D monolayer cell culturing and, thus, differentiate 2D samples from 3D and *in vivo* samples (**Figure 6**, red areas). Moreover, during the drug discovery process of treating cells with a test compound, in 2D, all of the cells are equally and highly exposed to the reagent and constituents of the media. In 3D cell culture, compounds and nutrients are subjected to diffusion gradients such as those seen in human tissues. Intuitively, there have been numerous studies that have shown differential compound efficacy when comparing the same cells grown in a 2D or 3D environment [22–24].

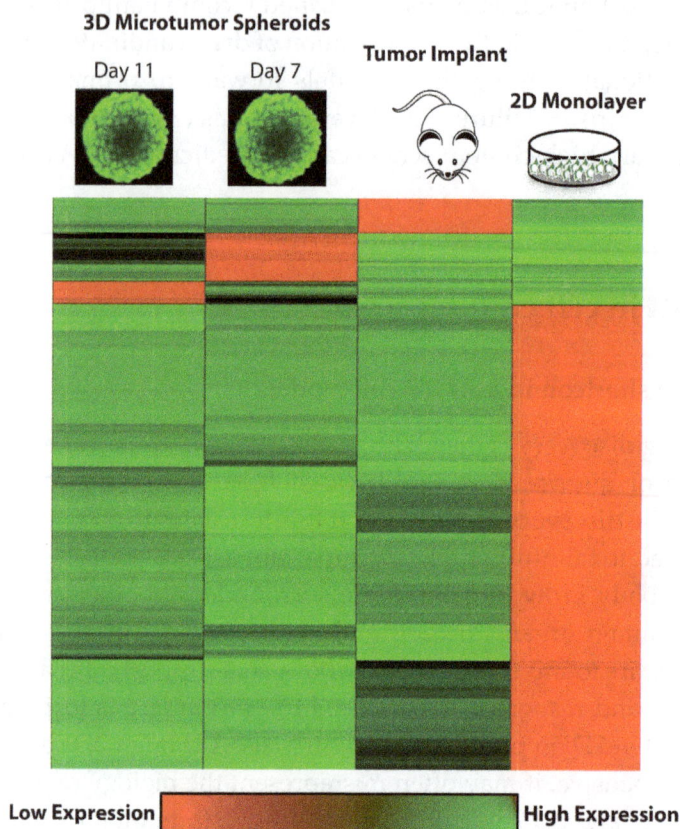

Figure 6. Comparison of melanoma cell gene expression in 2D, 3D and *in vivo*. RNAseq heat map of SK-MEL-30 human melanoma cells grown in 2D monolayer, 3D spheroids (day 7 and day 11 time points) and subcutaneous xenograft murine tumour implants. Hierarchical clustering of gene expression reveals similarities between 3D spheroid growth and *in vivo* growth. Two-dimensional monolayer growth results in massive downregulation of many genes (red areas).

As mentioned previously, phenotypic screening has been thoroughly integrated into modern drug discovery since its inception in the late 1990s. However, these screening efforts have mainly occurred in cells grown on plastic using a single parameter readout. Compounds and targets identified through 2D screens often do not translate their efficacies to *in vivo* animal models. Consequently, the use of 2D cell models puts into question the physiological relevance and translational applications of simple phenotypic screening models used in high-content drug discovery. Of course, nothing short of an animal model is expected to fully replicate *in vivo* biology, but more complex cell models growing in 3D may be able to address some of the shortcomings of conventional 2D cell models and may be more predictive of *in vivo* behaviour [25].

3.2. 3D cell models: development in academia and implementation in industry

The development of 3D and organotypic cell models has been rapidly expanding since the late 1990s. In particular, investigations at the Lawrence Berkeley National Laboratory by Mina Bissell and colleagues on breast cancer modelling revealed that 3D tumour cultures are more predictive of *in vivo* cellular behaviour than conventional 2D models, and these predictive powers typically extend to mouse xenograft tumour studies [26]. A steady but exponential increase in 3D cell model research has led to an abundance of literature on the subject over the last 10 years. In 2005, there were an estimated 135 papers reported in PubMed on "3D cell culture" and in 2015 that number jumped to 781 papers. Accordingly, there are currently several competing marketplaces for 3D cell culture reagents and *in vitro* tissue modelling services that did not exist 10 years ago. Consequently, there has been an overall recognition by academia and industry alike that modelling cells in 3D more closely mirrors organism biology and this has resulted in a revised understanding of the methods with which we practice drug discovery [25].

The adaptation of 3D cell models into high-content drug discovery has been relatively slow compared to their development and usage by academic investigators. There are several obvious reasons for the restricted employment of 3D models in pharmaceutical drug discovery, the most obvious being cost and labour. Three-dimensional screening platforms are relatively expensive compared to 2D platforms. The sources of the extra cost are often specialized 3D plates, ECM components and reagents required for multi-parametric phenotypic readouts; for example, antibodies or cell tracking dyes. Primarily, the main hurdle in adapting a 3D cell model to high-content PDD is technical logistics. Building a 3D screening platform is considerably more labour-intensive than a 2D cellular model. For large-scale screening efforts, the costs and labour associated with screening in 3D may be inhibitory. An important consideration when developing screening platforms for big pharma PDD is the workflow involved in the screen and its adaptability with automation. Something as straightforward and inconsequential as plating cells, for example, becomes considerably more complicated when transitioning from 2D to 3D. Traditional liquid handlers and cell dispensers that are used to create 2D cell models may not be compatible with the intended 3D model. For example, mixing and plating a cell/ECM suspension often requires precise temperature control that may not be possible using standard cell dispensers. Matrigel, a commonly used ECM in 3D tissue modelling, is viscous at cold temperatures but becomes rigid and fixed at 37°C. This means that the Matrigel/cell mixture must be kept cold during plating to ensure the matrix does not polymerize prematurely. Similarly, soft agar is another 3D matrix often used in tissue and tumour modelling and is viscous at warm temperatures but forms a rigid matrix when cooled to room temperature. Consequently, a soft agar/cell mixture must be kept warm during plating to prevent premature matrix formation. Translating these temperature-controlled logistical challenges to automation is not trivial. Although it is relatively straightforward to keep matrix/cell suspensions temperature-controlled in flasks or vessels, the temperature must be maintained during the movement of the mixture through the lines (tubing) of the instrument. Therefore, the lines must be jacketed in some fashion to maintain either a cold or warm temperature, depending on the matrix used, to prevent the mixture from polymerizing and clogging before reaching the dispenser. In a practical sense, this can be difficult to achieve, which is why many synthetic ECM reagents are currently being developed that do not require precise temperature control (discussed later). In a similar respect, cell dispensing instruments often use peristaltic pump devices to dispense cells. Peristaltic pumps can be abrupt in their action and may not be amenable to the careful dispensing required for a 3D cell model [25]. Consequently, a different type of cell-dispensing device, for example, a syringe-based system, may need to be engineered into the instrument to achieve the level of precision needed to create automated 3D cell models. In addition to modifications in automation, complex cell models that require feeder cells, gel matrices or scaffolding also provide for logistical challenges and complicated workflows [25]. Finally, complex 3D cell models often require long incubation times to manifest a particular phenotype or may require media changes or other manipulations needed to coax the model into the desired geometry. This type of precision may prove technically taxing compared with simpler 2D approaches, particularly in an automated format and at large scale [25].

An important aspect of complex and 3D cell models that is often overlooked in publications reporting their beneficial characteristics is that of variability. Two-dimensional monoculture screening platforms require few reagents for use and, subsequently, demonstrate minimal variance when assayed in PDD. Upon increasing the reagents involved for a complex assay (ECM, multiple different media or cell types), the variability is equally increased. The increasing number of variables that often accompany complex 3D cell models lead to an accumulation of potential variance. Further, 3D structures themselves, by virtue of their higher dimensional nature, are characterized by an increased level of heterogeneity than 2D systems [25]. With respect to assay readout, data acquisition of 3D structures is tremendously more challenging than for cells grown on plastic. This results in larger standard deviations for 3D cell models compared to 2D (personal observation). In order to overcome this inherent heterogeneity and account for the observed deviation, it becomes necessary to include more replicates within an assay. Including replicates within a primary screening assay results in a three to fourfold increase in cost or, alternatively, restricting the size of the library to be screened (discussed later).

In conclusion, 3D cell models are more expensive, technically challenging and labour-intensive to integrate into automated drug discovery at large scale compared to 2D models. However, in the discovery of novel targets and MoA that authentically represent patient disease biology, 3D models would seem to be superior to 2D models. Importantly, 3D models are often used to triage hit compounds from a 2D assay to an *in vivo* animal study. If that is the case, then those same gating 3D assays should be moved to the primary screening effort in order to reduce the quantity of false positive hits that investigators spend countless hours hunting down (**Figure 7A**). Another importance of primary screening in 3D is a reduction in time spent between the primary screen and the *in vivo* validation study. In this complicated climate of lengthy drug discovery programs, any shortening of timetables is extremely desirable and cost-effective. Most importantly, it has been observed that although many compounds may demonstrate comparable activities on cells grown in 2D or 3D, a large percentage of screened compounds (possibly 25%) may only demonstrate 3D-specific activity ([24] and reviewed in Ref. [27]). A benchmark example of this type of behaviour is Zalutumumab, an epidermal growth factor receptor (EGFR)-binding monoclonal antibody that only demonstrates efficacy in 3D *in vitro* and *in vivo* tumour models. These types of compounds would be missed under 2D screening conditions and may be important in addressing relevant disease biology (**Figure 7B**). Therefore, lately, it has become prudent for industrial drug discovery scientists to adapt into their high-content screening workflows, the 3D cell models created by academic researchers. The most apparent hurdle in this process is the miniaturization of complex and 3D cell models to accommodate a well of 384-well high-throughput screens (HTS) assay plate which is the size of two uncooked grains of rice. Ultimately, the goal is to progress from good models of tissue complexity and function into models that can be standardized and incorporated into high-content drug discovery [28].

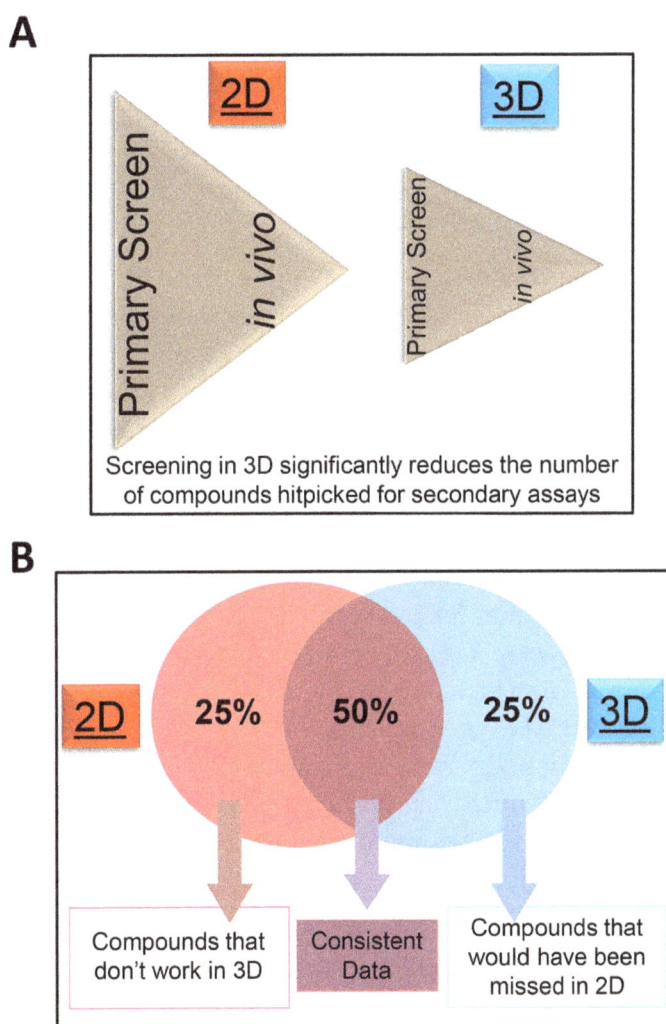

Figure 7. Three-dimensional screening may reduce drug development time and false positive rate. (A) Time between primary screening and *in vivo* modelling may be reduced using 3D primary HTS. (B) Primary 3D HTS may significantly reduce rate of false positives by as much as 25%.

4. Oncology research pioneers 3D cell modelling

4.1. An abbreviated history of 3D cell models in oncology research

It is estimated that within their lifetime, a person runs a 39.6% risk of being diagnosed with some form of cancer (National Cancer Institute, 2010–2012). This incredibly large patient population has driven the research and development functions in oncology faster and more furiously than any other disease field. In fact, 3D tumour modelling has been in constant use since the early 1970s. The multi-culture tumour spheroid (MCTS) model, which are tiny microtumours of self-assembled cancer cells, was developed in 1970 by Sutherland [29] and is still considered a crowning achievement in 3D tumour modelling. Similarly, the soft agar colony formation assay, which quantitates a cancer cell's anchorage-independent growth and self-renewal, was developed in 1976 by Courtenay [30] and continues to be widely employed as a gating assay for new experimental chemotherapeutics. Since that time 3D culture models developed for oncology research can be loosely grouped into three categories: (1) cells cultured as multicellular aggregates, (2) cells embedded within an extracellular matrix support (which might be natural or synthetic) and (3) cells cultured on inserts [28].

4.2. Screening the tumour microenvironment

Tumours (neoplasia) are complex tissue structures that harbour myriad cellular components similar to an organ. Neoplasia begins with transformed cancer cells that are often epithelial in origin. After the initial transformation and unrestricted cellular growth, cancer cells recruit neighbouring cells to feed tumour development and maintenance. These mesenchyme-derived cells, referred to as fibroblasts, then assume an activated state through the stimulation by cancer cells of fibroblast growth and secretory pathways. These activated "cancer-associated fibroblasts" (CAFs) further feed tumour development and actively participate in the recruit-ment of other types of cells to contribute to tumorigenesis. For example, CAFs are able to prevent immune recognition and T-cell-mediated tumour killing by secreting immunosup-pressive cytokines. These cytokines further blunt the innate immune response and stimulate the invasion of protumourigenic regulatory T-cells and M2 macrophages [31, 32]. Once tumours enlarge beyond 1–2 mm in diameter, they require oxygen to sustain viability because this is the maximal distance that oxygen and nutrients can diffuse without a blood supply [28]. CAFs stimulate neoangiogenesis by recruiting vascular endothelial cells and pericytes that form immature blood vessels, which then sustain tumour enlargement [33]. At this point, the tumour microenvironment (TME) has matured and contains many types of stromal cells (mesenchyme and hematopoietic) that all contribute to tumour survival and immune evasion (reviewed in Ref. [34]).

As one can imagine, accurately replicating the *in vivo* tumour microenvironment and all of its constituents in a Petri dish is not currently possible. That being said, there are elements of the tumour milieu that can be faithfully mimicked *in vitro* for the dissection of important cellular biology. The two most important features of *in vitro* tumour modelling are 3D growth and cell-to-cell communication. As mentioned earlier, there are currently three methods that dominate 3D tumour modelling: multicellular aggregates (spheroids), cancer cells embedded within an

ECM (colonies) and cancer cells cultured on inserts or transwells (skin, lung models and migration assays). Many of these complex models are at various stages of integration into high-content drug discovery.

4.3. The microtumour spheroid model

The spheroid model has gained a lot of popularity of late due to its tumour-like characteristics and ease of use in high-content screening. Spheroids can be thought of as tiny microtumours, in that they are self-assembled cancer structures organized into a hierarchical arrangement where cell-to-cell contacts create a 3D spherical structure. Spheroids often display properties and characteristics found in human tumours. For example, due to their complex structure, spheroids display gradients of oxygen and nutrients such that the outer shell of the spheroid contains rapidly proliferating cells (**Figure 8**). The proliferating shell surrounds a zone of quiescent cells, which further mantels a hypoxic area (**Figure 8**). The hypoxic zone is relatively large and results from a lack of oxygen penetration, mirroring *in vivo* avascular tumour physiology. In the centre of the spheroid is a necrotic core that contains dead or dying cells resulting from a large accumulation of metabolic waste products (e.g. lactate) and characterized as having low pH (**Figure 8**) [25]. The microtumour spheroid model has been widely adopted in high-content oncology drug discovery due to its emulating several important features of patient tumour biology that are not observed in cancer cells grown in 2D; namely, drug penetrance and hypoxia. Assaying for compound efficacy on cancer cells is equally as important as assaying for drug penetration; as one begets the other. Similarly, hypoxia-inducible factor (HIF) genes that respond to low oxygen concentration have been found to drive cancer stem cell behaviour in a variety of solid organ tumours [35]. There has been a barrage of literature around spheroids as models used in anticancer drug screening [36, 37], and further studies have shown how these models can be adapted to high-content drug discovery [38–40].

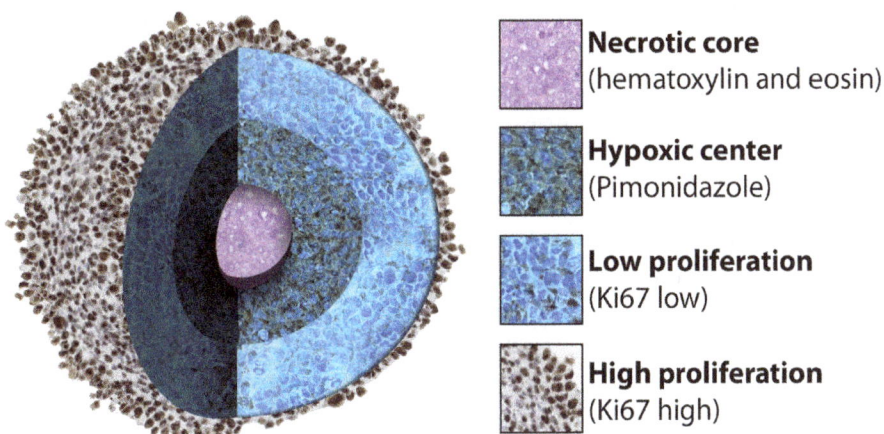

Necrotic core
(hematoxylin and eosin)

Hypoxic center
(Pimonidazole)

Low proliferation
(Ki67 low)

High proliferation
(Ki67 high)

Figure 8. The 3D microtumour spheroid cell model. Composite of immunohistochemistry images showing the necrotic core characterized by large lacunae of necrosis (haematoxylin and eosin stained), hypoxic area (pimonidazole duct staining) and zones of low proliferation (Ki67 low) and high proliferation (Ki67 high).

From a first-hand practical perspective, the spheroid platform represents an elegant biomimetic model for the identification of new molecular entities (NMEs) and MoAs. This is particularly true for finding targets and pathways that are only activated in a 3D context. There are several different methods that can be used to generate spheroids in 384-well high density format and they each have their respective benefits and liabilities. Numerous competing technologies exist for creating 384-well hanging drop spheroids (e.g. Perfecta 3D Hanging Drop Plates from 3D Biomatrix or the GravityPLUS System from InSphero), and these plates are easily adapted to high-content drug discovery [40, 41]. Similarly, low-attachment or round-bottom plates can be used to generate spheroids that are less technically cumbersome than the hanging drop system (e.g. 384-well Spheroid Plates from Corning or Ultra Low Attachment (ULA) Plates from SCIVAX). If cost is prohibitory, then ULA spheroid plates can be made in-house using standard U-bottom plates coated with 2-hydroxyethyl-methacrylate, which acts as a hydrogel in water and can induce 3D cellular aggregation [42]. Although spheroids are relatively easy to generate as far as 3D cellular structures go, they are more difficult to analyse effectively. The standard approach to quantifying changes in spheroid phenotype involves high-content confocal-based imaging. This can be achieved using antibodies that recognize a particular protein of interest or, more commonly, a chemical sensor that reports a biological phenotype (e.g. cell viability, cell death, caspase cleavage). The benefit of utilizing an imaging-based approach for the endpoint assay is that spheroid size and structure measurements can also be incorporated into the metrics to provide comprehensive and multi-parametric data [43]. However, as spheroids are several hundred micrometres thick and are rarely found on the exact same focal plane between wells, an autofocus feature on the imaging instrument is highly desirable. The other option is to assemble a Z-stack of images to address the focus problem, though that adds significant time and data storage issues to the readout process, particularly for large screens. Similarly, cell tracking using chemical sensors can be difficult to achieve over a week-long period of time as these dyes often degrade or become diluted with cell proliferation. What is increasingly being used for spheroid-based screens is a simple and straightforward CellTiter-Glo assay. CellTiter-Glo (Promega) is a luminescent viability assay that quantitates a cell's ATP and, thus, the amount of cells that are metabolically active. Recently, Promega developed a 3D-specific CellTiter-Glo 3D assay specifically designed for measuring spheroid viability, and this assay has been shown to be robust, sensitive and scalable to high-throughput screens [44]. Further, bioluminescent ATP detection assays offer relatively simple workflow and data analysis [44]. This may seem a low-tech readout for a high-tech cell model, but there are significantly fewer problems to overcome working with HTS bioluminescent viability assays compared to HTS imaging assays. Although you lose the benefit of a multi-parametric readout with CellTiter-Glo assays, the data are more robust and demonstrate less variance (personal observation).

4.4. HTS ECM assays

Another prevalent 3D screening platform used in oncology drug discovery is the colony formation assay that employs cells grown within an ECM. ECM strongly affects cellular organization and function and 3D cell models that incorporate ECM arguably help to better mimic *in vivo* biology, as they allow for cell-to-ECM interactions [45]. Though there are a variety of ECM-based assays employed in cancer cell modelling, the colony formation assay indisputably gets the most use. The assay enables the quantitation of a cell's anchorage-independent growth, through its ability to proliferate in 3D space. Additionally, as colonies are clonal resulting from the growth and proliferation of one particular cell, the colony formation assay also quantitates a sample's cancer stem cell population; as only cancer stem cells possess the property of self-renewal and clonal growth [46]. Historically, the 3D colony formation assay has been relegated to a secondary or tertiary screening platform by academics and industry scientists alike, where it has served as a gating step for moving forward new experimental therapeutics. Recently, investigators at Abbott Laboratories developed a soft agar colony formation assay that can be adapted to high-content screening, thereby bringing an important secondary assay to the forefront of primary phenotypic screening [47]. This 384-well 3D assay then opened the door for other big pharma screening projects such as the one by Sanofi-Aventis which involved screening 300,000 compounds on five different Kirsten RAt Sarcoma viral oncogene homologue (the most highly mutated and undruggable oncogene in human cancers) (KRAS)-dependent cancer cell lines grown in 3D ECM to identify pathways, targets or chemical matter with selective KRAS antitumor activity [48]. Researchers at Novartis have taken the 384-well colony formation assay even further, mixing normal colon fibroblasts together with colorectal carcinoma cells to achieve therapeutic indices of experimental test compounds [24]. The therapeutic index is a powerful metric for the simultaneous identification of a compound's therapeutic efficacy and potential toxicity.

There are a variety of matrix options commercially available for the design and implementation of HTS 3D ECM tumour assays. Soft agar is arguably the most common and least expensive ECM available and can be tittered to achieve the appropriate tensional force; an important characteristic when custom tailoring an ECM assay to different tissue and organ types. Matrigel (BD Biosciences), derived from the basement membranes of mouse sarcoma cells, is widely employed in HTS formats due to its easy-to-use thermal labile properties. However, Matrigel frequently contains cytokines and growth factors that demonstrate batch to batch inconsistencies which may result in unwanted or unpredictable variability [49]. In the past several years, there have been other ECM products developed for 3D assays that are similar to Matrigel such as ECL Cell Attachment Matrix (Millipore) and Geltrex (Life Sciences), which may offer advantages over conventional reagents. There is also a human placenta-derived ECM for 3D assays, HuBiogel (Vivo Biosciences), which has been shown to be a superior product for modelling human tissues due to its composition of collagens and laminins in biologically relevant proportions. Further, HuBiogel ECM is completely devoid of extraneous growth factors and cytokines, leading to more robust and reproducible 3D structure formation [50].

As opposed to naturally derived ECM substrates, there are also synthetic hydrogels that may be specifically engineered with chemical handles or attachment proteins to enable custom matrix conditions while still accounting for the heterogeneities present within the *in vivo* microenvironment. Chemically defined bioinert hydrogels can be customized with biomimetic and tissue-specific peptides to promote cell attachment and degradation in a robust format that may mitigate the need for naturally derived but ill-defined ECM [51]. These types of synthetic hydrogels are often not temperature labile and can be manipulated at room temperature, making them suitable reagents for use with automation in that there are no line- or tip-clogging problems to address. Some of these hydrogels (e.g. hyaluronic based hydrogels) can be systematically manipulated with distinct wavelengths of light (e.g. UV) to create custom ECM stiffness and density [52]. From a practical perspective, the synthetic ECM option may be more convenient for high-content approaches in that the cell/matrix mixture can be easily dispensed without the need for strict temperature control in the dispensing instrument. After plating, the ECM is cured through a quick exposure to UV light which solidifies the matrix and locks the cells in place. Synthetic ECM reagents are still currently in development by academic laboratories and have not yet been thoroughly integrated into high-content 3D drug discovery platforms.

4.5. Co-culture assays

Three-dimensional growth that addresses cell-to-ECM interactions is a key parameter for creating biomimetic tumour models. However, a parameter that is equally important to model in oncology drug discovery is cell-to-cell communication and this can only be accomplished through the use of co-cultures. Co-cultures are mixtures of two or more cell types within one assay with the goal of dissecting cellular crosstalk that may be important for modulating a particular phenotype. Co-culture assays are extremely relevant in oncology investigations in order to deconvolute biological signalling that occurs between different cell types within the TME. Cellular communication within the TME remains poorly understood and involves complex networks of secreted factors as well as direct ligand-to-receptor cellular interactions [53]. The most common co-culture assays used in oncology studies incorporate transformed cancer cells with cancer-associated fibroblasts (CAFs). The co-culturing of these two cell types often reveals important mechanisms by which fibroblasts can affect tumour cell behaviour and morphology. As CAFs often constitute the bulk of a tumour mass, it has become increasingly important to better understand their role in promoting and sustaining tumorigenesis, catalysing epithelial-to-mesenchymal transition (EMT; metastasis), suppressing the anti-tumorigenic immune response, and supporting drug resistance. In contrast to cancer cells, de novo acquisition of genetic mutations is less common in stromal cells than in malignant cells, so CAFs may be less prone to escape or resistance to a new therapy via genomic instability or epigenetic modifications. In the parlance of drug discovery, this means that a therapy targeting stromal components of the tumour may be more efficacious than targeting the transformed cells themselves and, moreover, may be more ubiquitously applied to many different types of neoplasia. Indeed a plethora of research investigating stromal targets for use in chemotherapy has surfaced during the last few years, supporting a more nuanced view of the contribution of stromal components to neoplastic transformation (reviewed in Ref. [54]). Prominently, CAFs have been shown to actively participate in tumour immunomodulation; CAF-secreted factors have been shown to suppress inflammation, antagonize T-cell invasion and recruit protumourigenic myeloid-derived cells to the tumour [32, 55].

There are a variety of methods to employ CAFs and tumour cells within the same 3D culture, and the approach is often dictated by the biological mechanism under investigation. For example, CAFs and tumour cells may be incorporated into a co-culture tumour spheroid to scrutinize direct cell-to-cell (ligand-receptor) communication between these two cell types. Alternatively, CAFs may be plated in 2D with cancer cells grown in 3D atop an ECM overlay, which may faithfully replicate secreted protein-based signalling between the different cell types. Using a genomics-based approach to study CAF-tumour cell interactions, genes may be knocked down using genomics reagents (siRNAs, virally-encoded shRNAs) within the CAFs and then assayed for a resulting phenotype within the cancer cells. This type of investigation may reveal CAF-specific genes or proteins involved in paracrine signalling that are crucial for tumour maintenance.

Continuing with the theme of tumour immunology, primary immune cells are also being used in co-culture with tumour cells to ascertain new mechanisms of immune-based targeted killing. Many of these elegant models employ 3D tumour spheroids and primary T-cells or natural killer (NK) cells in a high-content format to identify chemical reagents that can facilitate immune cell tumour recognition and killing [56]. These types of complex phenotypic screens may greatly expand the targeting space of conventional chemotherapeutics to include members of the tumour stroma such as CAFs and immune cells.

As with any complex phenotypic screening assay, co-culture systems present their own unique set of technical complications that must be overcome and optimized. Important considerations when developing a co-culture assay include the source of each cell type used (primary versus immortalized), ratios of cell types (biologically relevant proportions), length of culture time and data deconvolution. In terms of assay development, the cell culture media used may represent the most challenging hurdle. As different cell types require different types of media; glucose, amino acids, insulin, vitamins, serum, etc., all tittered to specific proportions, determining which media to use for a co-culture may require extensive empirical testing [53].

Another application of a co-culture assay is to identify potential and unwanted toxicity of a compound. In this example, fibroblasts and tumour cells may be mixed and assayed to obtain a therapeutic index of a test compound. Incorporating one target cell type with one normal cell type within the same screening well condenses the experimental workflow so that differential toxicity can be quantitated and used to triage hit compounds for further study [24]. This approach may complicate the primary assay but may also yield more therapeutically important data. In terms of assay readout, it may be crucial to distinguish between two different cell types. From an imaging- or flow cytometry-based perspective, this can be accomplished through the use of cell-specific reporter vectors; i.e. an enhanced green fluorescent protein (EGFP) reporter in tumour cells and a DsRed reporter in CAFs. A potentially easier approach is to label the different cell types with cell tracking dyes, though these types of chemical sensors tend to degrade and dilute over long time courses or may be swapped between different cells in close proximity (personal observation). Alternatively, if a luminescent screening platform is used, the different cell types may be engineered to express different forms of the luciferase enzyme. For example, tumour cells might express firefly luciferase and fibroblasts might express *Renilla* luciferase and a Dual-Glo Luciferase assay (Promega) can reveal differential luciferase signals and thus efficacy on tumour cells versus toxicity on fibroblasts. This approach requires a lengthy time of cell engineering but may produce robust and straightforward data for an HTS drug discovery effort. In short, the development of physiologically relevant co-culture assay systems for industrial drug discovery is challenging, but there are many technological innovations available to provide a scientific/technical tool box for the advancement of multi-culture primary phenotypic screening assays and improvement of early stage drug discovery [53].

4.6. Transwell models

The transwell plate system (also referred to as modified Boyden chambers) consists of a series of permeable supports inserted into wells of a cell culture plate. Cells can be plated in the lower chamber and/or the upper chamber, and the porous membrane can be exploited to study chemotaxis or cell migration, making it a versatile assay platform applicable to a variety of phenotypic screening experiments. In oncology research, the transwell system has been used to model the air-liquid interface for several different indications. Skin studies in particular are well modelled using the transwell system, where collagen and dermal fibroblasts are plated upon the insert and melanoma cells are layered on top. Melanoma cell invasion into the dermis is then quantitated by low-throughput methods such as histology of membrane cross sections. Transwell plates are also used for invasion assays of cancer cells. In this type of assay, cancer cells are plated in the top chamber over a layer of Matrigel (or another type of ECM) and a chemoattractant is added to the lower chamber to induce trans-membrane migration of cancer cells. Cancer cells that migrate through the ECM and invade the lower chamber can be quantitated by simple staining and counting [57]. Transwell plates are also used for immune cell migration assays. For example, in place of ECM, transwell inserts can be coated with vascular endothelial cells and immune cells (leukocytes) are plated on top. A chemoattractant is added to the lower chamber and transendothelial migration of immune cells is quantitated by cell staining and counting or, alternatively, antibody labelling for specific cell surface markers that distinguish the migrated population (e.g. T-cells or neutrophils). These methods can be modified to include tumour cells in the lower chamber and monocytes in the upper chamber. As monocytes migrate through the endothelial layer and invade the tumour cells they may differentiate into macrophages and become adherent, an enabling characteristic for quantitating invasion into tumour cell monolayers.

Transwell plates are typically used in low-throughput formats such as 12- or 24-well inserts. Currently, the most high density transwell plate is the 96-well plate made by Corning. The lack of high-content screenable formats has restricted the employment of transwell assays in phenotypic drug discovery. At present, the most common application of the 96-well transwell plate is for cell-based drug absorption assays [58]. In these approaches, CaCo-2 gut epithelial cells are plated as monolayers on the permeable inserts. Experimental test compounds are then added to this mock intestinal lining and permeability and transport characteristics of the compound are calculated. This component of Absorption, Distribution, Metabolism and Excretion (ADME)/tox (absorption, distribution, metabolism, and excretion) testing often determines whether a compound continues in the drug discovery process [59]. Development and implementation of a high density 384-well transwell plate may significantly expand phenotypic drug discovery for a range of different disease indications.

5. Complex phenotypic screening in other disease areas

5.1. Cellular differentiation and flow cytometry in PDD

Complex phenotypic screening assays do not necessarily require 3D cellular growth. Assuming the assay replicates an important and patient-relevant aspect of disease pathology, any multi-parametric phenotypic screen may be considered complex by comparative standards. For example, flow cytometry represents an unparalleled advance in the quantification of multi-parametric measurements on single cells. As mentioned earlier, one of the hallmarks of leukaemia is a block in differentiation. Rapid proliferation of immature, undifferentiated hematopoietic progenitor cells (blasts) leads to blast crisis which often takes the lives of acute myeloid leukaemia (AML) patients. Restoring the natural process of hematopoietic differentiation in these immature myeloid precursor cells usually results in a concomitant decrease in their proliferation. Flow cytometry is a technique well-suited to leukaemia research as identification of cell surface markers is the most common method used to characterize differentiated hematopoietic subtypes. Two leading researchers of leukaemia therapeutics, David Sykes and David Scadden at Massachusetts General Hospital, recently used a flow cytometry-based phenotypic screening approach to identify ML390, a compound identified from a collection of 330,000 compounds, which was able to restore differentiation of several human myeloid leukaemia cell models [43]. From a different assay perspective, flow cytometry can be used to multiplex viability readouts. Different cell types may be screened and then subjected to a fluorescent barcoding scheme where each cell type is given a unique tracker dye barcode, then pooled together and run through one flow cytometry readout (e.g. viability or apoptosis). This cellular barcoding method enables assay multiplexing and condensing multiple assays into one readout, which may often be the bottle neck of the screening experiment [44]. New technologies such as the high throughput sampler system (Becton Dickinson) and the HyperCyt platform (IntelliCyt) have recently enabled the application of 384- or 1536-well flow cytometry to large scale drug discovery phenotypic screening efforts [60]. Although flow cytometry is employed for single cell resolution, large particle flow cytometers (e.g. COPAS from Union Biometrica) are now capable of analysis and sorting of large macrocellular structures several hundred microns thick, such as spheroids [45]. Large particle flow cytometry may be ideally suited to the rapid analysis of spheroids or microtissues in suspension, a cumbersome task for high-content imagers [24].

The cellular differentiation phenotype may also be quantitated using an imaging-based approach, which is equally suited to high-content drug discovery. In a manner similar to flow cytometry, assayed cells are stained with antibodies that recognize cell surface markers, fixed and subjected to HTS imaging analysis. Imaging data are then analysed for the intensity and frequency of antibody staining and/or the co-localization of stem/differentiation markers. This method has been employed extensively by researchers in the field of regenerative medicine and has been shown to yield high quality robust data in primary HTS for compounds that expand hematopoietic stem cells (HSCs) for use in transplant therapy [61] or induces the selective differentiation of multipotent mesenchymal stem cells for cartilage repair [62].

5.2. Cell migration and wound repair

Cell migration and motility are important biological features common to different diseases. Cell migration assays are routinely used in the study of wound healing to identify therapeutics that can increase fibroblast, endothelial cell or epithelial cell migration. The so-called scratch assay is a convenient and inexpensive method that has been routinely employed for decades to study cell migration *in vitro* [63]. This method is based on the principle that, upon creation of an artificial gap (scratch) on a confluent cell monolayer, the cells on the edge of the scratch will move toward the opening, to close the scratch until new cell-to-cell contacts are established [64]. The scratch assay is overly simple and can be accomplished using common and inexpensive supplies routinely found in most cell culture laboratories. Employing an imaging-based readout to the assay, the width of the scratch is measured at the beginning of the assay and then at subsequent intervals throughout the assay until the scratch is closed. The scratch assay can be integrated into high-content wound healing screens for the discovery and validation of small molecule leads and other perturbagens that affect cell migration [65]. However, at smaller screenable formats such as 384- or 1536-well, making scratches in wells becomes much more difficult to achieve with consistency and reproducibility (**Figure 9A**) which is why other migration-assaying technologies have been developed.

Cell migration and motility also play vital roles in the process of tumour metastasis. However, in this case, the goal is the identification of anti-migratory agents that might be used in the clinic to restrict metastasis. Due to the inherent heterogeneity of the scratches made during an HTS scratch assay, a technology slightly more sophisticated was developed that is more robust during high-content imaging. The Oris™ Pro assay system (Platypus Technologies) is a novel, multi-parametric cell migration assay that is available in 384-well format and is fully compatible with automated microscopy and high-content screening [66]. This technology employs a circular plug in the centre of the well around which cells adhere and grow. The plug then dissolves revealing a perfectly centred circular zone of no cell growth. High-content imaging measures the diameter of the circle at day 1 and all subsequent time points until cells grow over the zone. The benefit of this assay over the scratch assay in studying metastasis is that cells are not physically disrupted and sheared as they would be in the scratch assay which is a more appropriate model of wound generation/repair. The Oris™ platform was recently used to identify compounds that inhibit cell motility in human breast cancer cells in an HTS format [66]. A similar type of assay platform was developed by collaborating biologists and engineers and consists of a 384-well silicon plug system that fits into the assay plate [67]. As opposed to the Oris™ system, the ZonEx system demonstrates robust consistency and reproducibility between wells (**Figure 9B**). Further, it is a reusable technology in contrast to the Oris™ system that is a one-use product [67].

Most currently available migration and motility assays exist only for 2D cell culturing, which may not necessarily mimic the complex mechanical and biochemical interplay between various cells and the ECM microenvironment that occurs in human patients. To address invasion dynamics in 3D culture, a multi-parametric 3D HTS platform for cell motility and invasion was recently developed [68]. In this vertical gel invasion assay, cells are seeded on top of a collagen matrix and their migration/invasion into the gel is quantitated from a Z-stack taken with a laser-scanning confocal microscope. This approach is more biomimetic than traditional 2D scratch and zone exclusion assays and may reveal important perturbagens of 3D cell migration, for example, integrin-modulating agents. Unfortunately, a drawback to this approach is the requirement of Z-stack image assembly at multiple time points which can result in terabytes or even petabytes of data storage for a large scale compound screen.

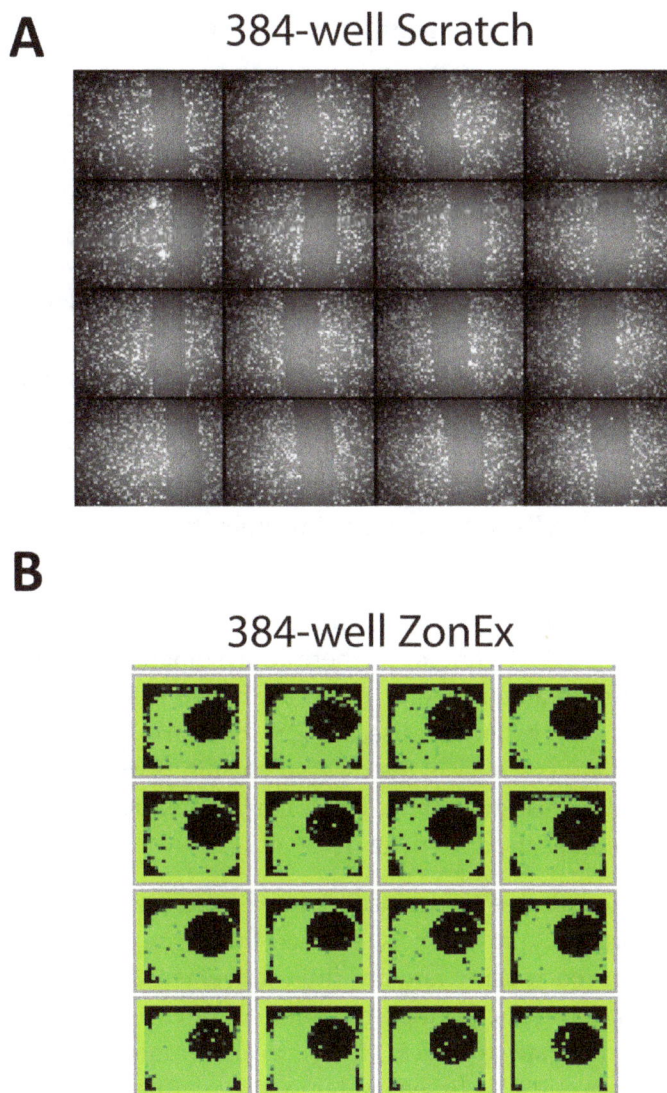

A   384-well Scratch

B   384-well ZonEx

Figure 9. Comparison of two HTS cell migration assays. (A) The standard scratch assay in 384-well format demonstrates wide variability of the position and width of the scratch, resulting in poor reproducibility. (B) The ZonEx assay makes perfectly circular zones of the same dimensions and at the same place in every well of a 384-well plate, yielding robust data. *Images courtesy of Nicholas Ng and Orzala Sharif.*

Overall, there are a wide variety of different assays available to screen for modulators of cell migration and motility either in 2D or 3D (reviewed in Ref. [69]). The different assay platforms range from simple and inexpensive to technically demanding and costly and the suitability of a particular method may be limited when considering a specific research question [69]. However, the continued integration of these sophisticated and complex phenotypic screening platforms into industrial drug discovery may significantly advance the quality of pro- and anti-migratory therapeutics progressed to the clinic.

6. Future outlook of complex phenotypic screening

The goal of phenotypic screening is the identification of new molecular entities, targets and mechanisms that can be exploited to create better disease-specific therapeutics. As opposed to target-based screening that occurs in an artificial biochemical environment, phenotypic screening takes advantage of the native cellular environment, a necessary quality when assaying for novel disease biology. Improving upon this, complex phenotypic screening expands the cellular environment further to include the extracellular environment, which actively participates in cellular disease pathology. Three-dimensional and complex HTS is relatively new to industrial drug discovery and has yet to prove its impact in big pharma. Although a wide range of products, technologies and services are currently available to facilitate 3D/complex HTS drug discovery, there are three key components that must be incorporated and addressed to ensure maximum success for future screening endeavours: (1) screening disease-relevant cells, (2) incorporating microfluidics and (3) decreasing assay capacity.

First, induced pluripotent stem cells (iPS) or patient-derived primary cells should be used for screening. Advancements in iPS technology, where adult somatic cells are reprogrammed into a pluripotent state similar to an embryonic stem cell, have provided a renewable source for relevant cell types for a wide variety of diseases [25]. Similarly, patient-derived iPS cells are able to recapitulate the characteristics of the disease phenotype from a patient and may open the door for personalized disease modelling. This, in turn, should improve the predictive value of complex *in vitro* cell models used for drug discovery [25].

Second, converting static cultures to perfused cultures using microfluidics devices will be crucial for optimizing organotypic cell models. Microfluidics represents a potentially revolutionary cell culturing approach using laminar fluid movement that better mimics the physiology of living tissues and organs. Further, microfluidic devices can support 3D cell culture making them excellent surrogates for the *in vivo* extracellular microenvironment (reviewed in Ref. [70]). However, microfluidics-based cell models require more miniaturization and engineering to create HTS-compatible assay platforms that incorporate active perfusion of media, growth supplements and test reagents. Microfluidics devices are not currently adapted into drug discovery screening and this may be largely due to the need for peristaltic pumps and other valves and mixers that accompany the plates. The ONIX system developed by CellASIC® incorporates a clever workaround for pumps, instead using gravity and surface tension to facilitate fluid flow through the plate. Continuous perfusion of the wells is maintained by refilling the inlet and emptying the outlet [71]. Although these plates can currently only accommodate 32 wells, the concept of fluid flow without the need for active pumping is

a great technological advancement for the field. Another microfluidics plate which does not require use of a pump is the Iuvo Microchannel 5250 system (BellBrook Labs) that uses a passive pumping technology to move fluid between two inlets connected by a channel. Iuvo plates come in 192-channel formats making them potentially useful for high-content phenotypic screening. Early stage drug discovery could greatly benefit from the integration of microfluidic tools into primary platforms which, in most cases, represents an improvement upon existing screening technologies [25].

Third, shifting the current screening paradigm from assay capacity to assay relevance may improve the quality of new therapeutics. Technological advancements that facilitate screening of complex cell models will undoubtedly be associated with a lower throughput than current simple 2D cell models. This translates to fewer 1536-well formatted cell models and, thus, smaller compound and reagent libraries that can be screened. Smaller focused screens sample chemical space instead of blanket coverage, but provide more insightful information when combined with multi-parametric, multi-time point assays [25]. By employing the concept of mechanistically informed drug discovery, smaller, more focused screens that allow multiplexed dynamic readouts may produce data of much higher quality with respect to predicted patient response [25], and this should ultimately result in the discovery of more successful therapeutics.

7. Conclusion

During the process of industrial drug discovery where new therapeutics are being tested in cell-based phenotypic screening assays, the culture methods used should mimic the most natural *in vivo* representative form possible [45]. In order to maximize success in the current drug development space, new technologies and methods must continue to evolve. Emerging phenotypic assay platforms must be critically compared and evaluated and, most importantly, must share extensive likeness with real tissue or tumour architecture. Incorporating 3D and complex phenotypic cellular assays into high-content drug discovery screening may effectively reduce the false positive hit rate, accelerate preclinical *in vivo* animal disease model studies and ultimately yield more efficacious and less toxic treatments for disease.

Author details

Shane R. Horman

Address all correspondence to: shorman@gnf.org

Advanced Assays, Genomics Institute of the Novartis Research Foundation, San Diego, CA, USA

References

[1] Eder J, Sedrani R, Wiesmann C. The discovery of first-in-class drugs: origins and evolution. Nature Reviews Drug Discovery. 2014 Aug;13(8):577–87. doi:10.1038/nrd4336

[2] Ehrlich P, Hata S. Die Experimentelle Chemotherapie der Spirilosen. Berlin: Julius Springer; 1910.

[3] Aminov RI. A brief history of the antibiotic era: lessons learned and challenges for the future. Frontiers in Microbiology. 2010;1:134. doi:10.3389/fmicb.2010.00134

[4] Harrison RG, Greenman MJ, Mall FP, Jackson CM. Observations on the living developing nerve fiber. The Anatomical Record. 1907;1(5):116–8.doi: 10.1002/ar.1090010503

[5] Scherer WF, Syverton JT, Gey GO. Studies on the propagation in vitro of poliomyelitis viruses. IV. Viral multiplication in a stable strain of human malignant epithelial cells (strain HeLa) derived from an epidermoid carcinoma of the cervix. The Journal of Experimental Medicine. 1953 May;97(5):695–710

[6] Moffat JG, Rudolph J, Bailey D. Phenotypic screening in cancer drug discovery – past, present and future. Nature Reviews Drug Discovery. 2014 Aug;13(8):588–602. doi: 10.1038/nrd4366

[7] Garraway LA, Lander ES. Lessons from the cancer genome. Cell. 2013 Mar 28;153(1): 17–37. doi:10.1016/j.cell.2013.03.002

[8] Swinney DC. Phenotypic vs. target-based drug discovery for first-in-class medicines. Clinical Pharmacology and Therapeutics. 2013 Apr;93(4):299–301. doi:10.1038/clpt. 2012.236

[9] Nowell PC, Hungerford D. A minute chromosome in chronic granulocytic leukemia. Science. 1960;132(3438):1497. doi:10.1126/science.132.3438.1488

[10] Rowley JD. Letter: A new consistent chromosomal abnormality in chronic myelogenous leukaemia identified by quinacrine fluorescence and Giemsa staining. Nature. 1973 Jun 1;243(5405):290–3

[11] Shtivelman E, Lifshitz B, Gale RP, Canaani E. Fused transcript of abl and bcr genes in chronic myelogenous leukaemia. Nature. 1985 Jun 13–19;315(6020):550–4

[12] Druker BJ, Lydon NB. Lessons learned from the development of an abl tyrosine kinase inhibitor for chronic myelogenous leukemia. The Journal of Clinical Investigation. 2000 Jan;105(1):3–7. doi:10.1172/JCI9083

[13] Friend C, Scher W, Holland JG, Sato T. Hemoglobin synthesis in murine virus-induced leukemic cells in vitro: stimulation of erythroid differentiation by dimethyl sulfoxide. Proceedings of the National Academy of Sciences of the United States of America. 1971 Feb;68(2):378–82

[14] Richon VM, Emiliani S, Verdin E, Webb Y, Breslow R, Rifkind RA, et al. A class of hybrid polar inducers of transformed cell differentiation inhibits histone deacetylases. Proceedings of the National Academy of Sciences of the United States of America. 1998 Mar 17;95(6):3003–7

[15] Marks PA, Breslow R. Dimethyl sulfoxide to vorinostat: development of this histone deacetylase inhibitor as an anticancer drug. Nature Biotechnology. 2007 Jan;25(1):84–90. doi:10.1038/nbt1272

[16] Hart CP. Finding the target after screening the phenotype. Drug Discovery Today. 2005 Apr 1;10(7):513–9. doi:10.1016/S1359–6446(05)03415-X

[17] Katayama H, Oda Y. Chemical proteomics for drug discovery based on compound-immobilized affinity chromatography. Journal of Chromatography B, Analytical Technologies in the Biomedical and Life Sciences. 2007 Aug;855(1):21–7. doi:10.1016/j.jchromb.2006.12.047

[18] King FJ, Selinger, DW, Mapa, FA, Janes, J, Wu, H, Smith, TR, Wang, Q, Niyomrattana-kitand, P, Sipes, DG, Brinker, A, Porter, JA and Myer, VE. Pathway reporter assays reveal small molecule mechanisms of action. Journal of Laboratory Automation. 2009;14(6):374–82. doi:10.1016/j.jala.2009.08.001

[19] O'Brien LE, Zegers MM, Mostov KE. Opinion: Building epithelial architecture: insights from three-dimensional culture models. Nature Reviews Molecular Cell Biology. 2002 Jul;3(7):531–7. doi:10.1038/nrm859

[20] Bissell MJ, Radisky D. Putting tumours in context. Nature Reviews Cancer. 2001 Oct; 1(1):46–54. doi:10.1038/35094059

[21] Smalley KS, Lioni M, Herlyn M. Life isn't flat: taking cancer biology to the next dimension. In vitro Cellular and Developmental Biology Animal. 2006 Sep-Oct;42(8–9):242–7. doi:10.1290/0604027.1

[22] Lovitt CJ, Shelper TB, Avery VM. Miniaturized three-dimensional cancer model for drug evaluation. Assay and Drug Development Technologies. 2013 Sep;11(7):435–48. doi:10.1089/adt.2012.483

[23] Hongisto V, Jernstrom S, Fey V, Mpindi JP, Kleivi Sahlberg K, Kallioniemi O, et al. High-throughput 3D screening reveals differences in drug sensitivities between culture models of JIMT1 breast cancer cells. PLoS One. 2013;8(10):e77232. doi:10.1371/journal.pone.0077232

[24] Horman SR, To J, Orth AP. An HTS-compatible 3D colony formation assay to identify tumor-specific chemotherapeutics. Journal of Biomolecular Screening. 2013 Dec;18(10): 1298–308. doi:10.1177/1087057113499405

[25] Horman SR, Hogan C, Delos Reyes K, Lo F, Antczak C. Challenges and opportunities toward enabling phenotypic screening of complex and 3D cell models. Future Medicinal Chemistry. 2015;7(4):513–25. doi:10.4155/fmc.14.163

[26] Weaver VM, Petersen OW, Wang F, Larabell CA, Briand P, Damsky C, et al. Reversion of the malignant phenotype of human breast cells in three-dimensional culture and in vivo by integrin blocking antibodies. The Journal of Cell Biology. 1997 Apr 7;137(1): 231–45

[27] Edmondson R, Broglie JJ, Adcock AF, Yang L. Three-dimensional cell culture systems and their applications in drug discovery and cell-based biosensors. Assay and Drug Development Technologies. 2014 May;12(4):207–18. doi:10.1089/adt.2014.573

[28] Kimlin LC, Casagrande G, Virador VM. In vitro three-dimensional (3D) models in cancer research: an update. Molecular Carcinogenesis. 2013 Mar;52(3):167–82. doi: 10.1002/mc.21844

[29] Sutherland RM, Inch WR, McCredie JA, Kruuv J. A multi-component radiation survival curve using an in vitro tumour model. International Journal of Radiation Biology and Related Studies in Physics, Chemistry, and Medicine. 1970;18(5):491–5

[30] Courtenay VD. A soft agar colony assay for Lewis lung tumour and B16 melanoma taken directly from the mouse. British Journal of Cancer. 1976 Jul;34(1):39–45

[31] Ham M, Moon A. Inflammatory and microenvironmental factors involved in breast cancer progression. Archives of Pharmacal Research. 2013 Dec;36(12):1419–31. doi: 10.1007/s12272-013-0271-7

[32] De Monte L, Reni M, Tassi E, Clavenna D, Papa I, Recalde H, et al. Intratumor T helper type 2 cell infiltrate correlates with cancer-associated fibroblast thymic stromal lymphopoietin production and reduced survival in pancreatic cancer. The Journal of Experimental Medicine. 2011 Mar 14;208(3):469–78. doi:10.1084/jem.20101876

[33] Orimo A, Gupta PB, Sgroi DC, Arenzana-Seisdedos F, Delaunay T, Naeem R, et al. Stromal fibroblasts present in invasive human breast carcinomas promote tumor growth and angiogenesis through elevated SDF-1/CXCL12 secretion. Cell. 2005 May 6;121(3):335–48. doi:10.1016/j.cell.2005.02.034

[34] Hanahan D, Weinberg RA. Hallmarks of cancer: the next generation. Cell. 2011 Mar 4;144(5):646–74. doi:10.1016/j.cell.2011.02.013

[35] Menrad H, Werno C, Schmid T, Copanaki E, Deller T, Dehne N, et al. Roles of hypoxia-inducible factor-1alpha (HIF-1alpha) versus HIF-2alpha in the survival of hepatocellular tumor spheroids. Hepatology. 2010 Jun;51(6):2183–92. doi:10.1002/hep.23597

[36] Kunz-Schughart LA, Freyer JP, Hofstaedter F, Ebner R. The use of 3-D cultures for high-throughput screening: the multicellular spheroid model. Journal of Biomolecular Screening. 2004 Jun;9(4):273–85. doi:10.1177/1087057104265040

[37] Hirschhaeuser F, Menne H, Dittfeld C, West J, Mueller-Klieser W, Kunz-Schughart LA. Multicellular tumor spheroids: an underestimated tool is catching up again. Journal of Biotechnology. 2010 Jul 1;148(1):3–15. doi:10.1016/j.jbiotec.2010.01.012

[38] LaBarbera DV, Reid BG, Yoo BH. The multicellular tumor spheroid model for high-throughput cancer drug discovery. Expert Opinion on Drug Discovery. 2012 Sep;7(9): 819–30. doi:10.1517/17460441.2012.708334

[39] Ho WY, Yeap SK, Ho CL, Rahim RA, Alitheen NB. Development of multicellular tumor spheroid (MCTS) culture from breast cancer cell and a high throughput screening method using the MTT assay. PLoS One. 2012;7(9):e44640. doi:10.1371/journal.pone. 0044640

[40] Horman SR, To J, Orth AP, Slawny N, Cuddihy MJ, Caracino D. High-content analysis of three-dimensional tumor spheroids: investigating signaling pathways using small hairpin RNA. Nature Methods. 2013 10//print;10(10). 40: V–Vi. doi:10.1038/nmeth.f.370

[41] Tung YC, Hsiao AY, Allen SG, Torisawa YS, Ho M, Takayama S. High-throughput 3D spheroid culture and drug testing using a 384 hanging drop array. The Analyst. 2011 Feb 7;136(3):473–8. doi:10.1039/c0an00609b

[42] Tong JZ, De Lagausie P, Furlan V, Cresteil T, Bernard O, Alvarez F. Long-term culture of adult rat hepatocyte spheroids. Experimental Cell Research. 1992 Jun; 200(2):326–32

[43] Li L, Zhou Q, Voss TC, Quick KL, LaBarbera DV. High-throughput imaging: Focusing in on drug discovery in 3D. Methods. 2016 Mar 1;96:97–102. doi:10.1016/j.ymeth. 2015.11.013

[44] Kijanska M, Kelm J. In vitro 3D spheroids and microtissues: ATP-based cell viability and toxicity assays. In: Sittampalam GS, Coussens NP, Nelson H, Arkin M, Auld D, Austin C, et al., editors. Assay Guidance Manual. Bethesda, MD, NIH-NCATS: the National Center for Advancing Translational Sciences. 2004.

[45] Breslin S, O'Driscoll L. Three-dimensional cell culture: the missing link in drug discovery. Drug Discovery Today. 2013 Mar;18(5–6):240–9. doi:10.1016/j.drudis. 2012.10.003

[46] Hamburger AW, Salmon SE. Primary bioassay of human tumor stem cells. Science. 1977 Jul 29;197(4302):461–3

[47] Anderson SN, Towne DL, Burns DJ, Warrior U. A high-throughput soft agar assay for identification of anticancer compound. Journal of Biomolecular Screening. 2007 Oct; 12(7):938–45. doi:10.1177/1087057107306130

[48] Koundinya M, Sudhalter J, Courjaud A, Lionne B, Touyer G, Bonnet L, et al. Clonogenic 3D high throughput screening in mutant KRAS dependent cancer cells – a chemogenomic approach. In: Proceedings of the 104th Annual Meeting of the American Association for Cancer Research. 2013;73:1. doi:10.1158/1538–7445.AM2013-2243

[49] Hughes CS, Postovit LM, Lajoie GA. Matrigel: a complex protein mixture required for optimal growth of cell culture. Proteomics. 2010 May;10(9):1886–90. doi:10.1002/ pmic.200900758

[50] Yuan K, Kucik D, Singh RK, Listinsky CM, Listinsky JJ, Siegal GP. Alterations in human breast cancer adhesion-motility in response to changes in cell surface glycoproteins displaying alpha-L-fucose moieties. International Journal of Oncology. 2008 Apr;32(4): 797–807

[51] Belair DG, Schwartz MP, Knudsen T, Murphy WL. Human iPSC-derived endothelial cell sprouting assay in synthetic hydrogel arrays. Acta Biomaterialia. 2016 May 13. doi: 10.1016/j.actbio.2016.05.020

[52] Rape AD, Zibinsky M, Murthy N, Kumar S. A synthetic hydrogel for the high-throughput study of cell-ECM interactions. Nature Communications. 2015;6:8129. doi: 10.1038/ncomms9129

[53] Berg, EL, Hsu YC, Lee JA. Consideration of the cellular microenvironment: physiolog-ically relevant co-culture systems in drug discovery. Advanced Drug Delivery Reviews. 2014 Apr;69–70:190–204. doi:10.1016/j.addr.2014.01.013

[54] Junttila MR, de Sauvage FJ. Influence of tumour micro-environment heterogeneity on therapeutic response. Nature. 2013 Sep 19;501(7467):346–54. doi:10.1038/nature12626

[55] Erez N, Truitt M, Olson P, Arron ST, Hanahan D. Cancer-associated fibroblasts are activated in incipient neoplasia to orchestrate tumor-promoting inflammation in an NF-kappaB-dependent manner. Cancer Cell. 2010 Feb 17;17(2):135–47. doi:10.1016/j.ccr. 2009.12.041

[56] Giannattasio A, Weil S, Kloess S, Ansari N, Stelzer EH, Cerwenka A, et al. Cytotoxicity and infiltration of human NK cells in in vivo-like tumor spheroids. BMC Cancer. 2015;15:351. doi:10.1186/s12885-015-1321-y

[57] Furukawa S, Soeda S, Kiko Y, Suzuki O, Hashimoto Y, Watanabe T, et al. MCP-1 promotes invasion and adhesion of human ovarian cancer cells. Anticancer Research. 2013 Nov;33(11):4785–90

[58] Marino AM, Yarde M, Patel H, Chong S, Balimane PV. Validation of the 96 well Caco-2 cell culture model for high throughput permeability assessment of discovery com-pounds. International Journal of Pharmaceutics. 2005 Jun 13;297(1–2):235–41. doi: 10.1016/j.ijpharm.2005.03.008

[59] Larson B, Banks P, Sherman H, Rothenberg M. Automation of cell-based drug absorp-tion assays in 96-well format using permeable support systems. Journal of Laboratory Automation. 2012 Jun;17(3):222–32. doi:10.1177/2211068211428190

[60] Joslin J, Gilligan J, Anderson P, Sharif O, Garcia C, Trussell C, et al. Development of a fully automated ultra-high-throughput flow cytometry screening system to enable novel drug discovery. SLAS: Society for Laboratory Automation and Screening. 2014:70

[61] Boitano AE, Wang J, Romeo R, Bouchez LC, Parker AE, Sutton SE, et al. Aryl hydro-carbon receptor antagonists promote the expansion of human hematopoietic stem cells. Science. 2010 Sep 10;329(5997):1345–8. doi:10.1126/science.1191536

[62] Johnson K, Zhu S, Tremblay MS, Payette JN, Wang J, Bouchez LC, et al. A stem cell-based approach to cartilage repair. Science. 2012 May 11;336(6082):717–21. doi:10.1126/science.1215157

[63] Todaro GJ, Lazar GK, Green H. The initiation of cell division in a contact-inhibited mammalian cell line. Journal of Cellular Physiology. 1965 Dec;66(3):325–33

[64] Liang CC, Park AY, Guan JL. In vitro scratch assay: a convenient and inexpensive method for analysis of cell migration in vitro. Nature Protocols. 2007;2(2):329–33. doi:10.1038/nprot.2007.30

[65] Yarrow JC, Perlman ZE, Westwood NJ, Mitchison TJ. A high-throughput cell migration assay using scratch wound healing, a comparison of image-based readout methods. BMC Biotechnology. 2004 Sep 9;4:21. doi:10.1186/1472-6750-4-21

[66] Joy ME, Vollmer LL, Hulkower K, Stern AM, Peterson CK, Boltz RC, et al. A high-content, multiplexed screen in human breast cancer cells identifies profilin-1 inducers with anti-migratory activities. PLoS One. 2014;9(2):e88350. doi:10.1371/journal.pone.0088350

[67] Sharif O, Chang J, Wilson AJ, Borboa A, Gardiner E. ZonEx: A novel device to enable high throughput cell migration assays [seminar]. LEADs Meeting, San Diego, California, 2013.

[68] Burgstaller G, Oehrle B, Koch I, Lindner M, Eickelberg O. Multiplex profiling of cellular invasion in 3D cell culture models. PLoS One. 2013;8(5):e63121. doi:10.1371/journal.pone.0063121

[69] Kramer N, Walzl A, Unger C, Rosner M, Krupitza G, Hengstschlager M, et al. In vitro cell migration and invasion assays. Mutation Research. 2013 Jan-Mar;752(1):10–24. doi:10.1016/j.mrrev.2012.08.001

[70] Huh D, Hamilton GA, Ingber DE. From 3D cell culture to organs-on-chips. Trends in Cell Biology. 2011 Dec;21(12):745–54. doi:10.1016/j.tcb.2011.09.005

[71] Chen SY, Hung PJ, Lee PJ. Microfluidic array for three-dimensional perfusion culture of human mammary epithelial cells. Biomedical Microdevices. 2011 Aug;13(4):753–8. doi:10.1007/s10544-011-9545-3

7

QbD Implementation in Biotechnological Product Development Studies

Buket Aksu, Ali Demir Sezer, Gizem Yeğen and
Lale Kuşçu

Additional information is available at the end of the chapter

Abstract

Biotechnological drug development is an extensive area still growing and coming into prominence day by day. Since biotechnological product manufacturing is irreversible, highly expensive, and contains so many critical parameters throughout the process, quality control tests applied to the finished product become inefficacious; therefore, maintaining predefined quality is crucial. Quality by Design (QbD), a systematic approach, is designing and optimizing of formulation and production processes in order to provide a predefined product quality by following a risk and scientific-based path. Determining the critical variables for biotechnological products and their manufacturing via risk assessment is the first and most vital stage of QbD approach, before exploring the multivariate relations among the independent and dependent critical variables by mathematical modeling with the assistive technologies. Response Surface Method (RSM), Artificial Neural Network (ANN), and Genetic Algorithm (GA) are some of the assistive technologies used to perform mathematical modeling. After modeling, additional knowledge is vested and this provides the chance to find a range in which the product quality is always ensured, called as "Design space". So, product quality is procured all along the process by keeping the critical variables under control with less effort, money, and mistakes.

Keywords: biotechnology, production, QbD, ICH

1. Introduction

Pharmaceutical manufacturing is a complicated process from formulation to the final product. It is crucial to understand that multivariate interactions between raw materials and process conditions take place in the manufacturing process to ensure processability and product quality. Despite continuous innovations in the pharmaceutical industry for developing new, futuristic drug products, there have been a repeated set back due to low quality and manufacturing standards. The studies and tests required to deliver a new drug to end-users takes up to 15 years, and cost over 800 million $. Even after a drug is invented, due to the proven incapability for its safe manufacture in a large scale and incompliance with the relevant specifications, its development may fail. The approval process duration and the requirement to start over a development cycle because of any changes resulted from stalemates have both given rise to concerns for decades. Nowadays it is known that this process, involving a significant amount of paperwork for evaluation and approval of new product submissions, is slow and overwhelming and causes excessive delays [1].

2. ICH Guidelines: objectives and history

Traditional pharmaceutical manufacturing is accomplished by using batch processing with quality control testing conducted on samples of the finished product. Despite the loss of too many products and investment, this conventional approach has been considered sufficient in providing quality pharmaceuticals to the public for many years. However, innovation in product and process development, process analysis, and process control can provide significant opportunities for improving pharmaceutical development, manufacturing, and quality assurance [2].

Process change is an expected aspect of pharmaceutical manufacturing. To keep pace with advancing technologies and improvements in the manufacturing process, many process changes are made resulting from increased process knowledge. When a product is first approved, its manufacturing process represents the current technology standard for manufacturing and follows the current standards for regulatory compliance. After approval, the approved process may need to be modified due to changes in market demand, technological advances, manufacturing standards, raw materials sourcing, or manufacturing experience. Traditionally, postapproval changes require regulatory agency approval before implementation. The increasing number of new products in addition to the number of marketed products seeking postapproval changes has placed a significant burden on the government and industry to submit and review data to comply with existing requirements. Thus, we need to identify a path forward that will enhance substantial product and process knowledge using risk assessment tools and quality systems to ensure product safety and efficacy [3].

Because of all these reasons, the drug industry experienced major developments in production information, quality management systems, and risk management in recent years. The industry developed modern production tools that can assist in ensuring product quality [1]. Thus, Food and Drug Administration (FDA) introduced the amendments in the current Good Manufacturing Practices (cGMP) to the pharmaceutical industry, to improve and modernize the rules that regulate the pharmaceutical product manufacturing and product quality since 2002, in accordance with the developments in the twenty-first century. International Conference on

Harmonization (ICH) is a forum for registered institutions and experts from the pharmaceutical industries in the United States (US), Japan, and European Union to harmonize the technical requirements for pharmaceutical products in three regions. It provides up-to-date guidelines bringing a new approach called Quality by Design (QbD) to the pharmaceutical industry [4]. The new series of quality guidelines (Q8, Q9, Q10, and Q11) were published by ICH regarding the QbD concept which was introduced into the FDA's chemistry, manufacturing, and controls (CMC) review process in 2004 [5]. Subsequently, in 2005, the guideline Q8 "pharmaceutical development" of the International Conference on Harmonization (ICH), which focused on the content of the module 3.2.P.2 of the common technical document (CTD), was published to present a roadmap for a proper QbD implementation [1]. These improvements have added new dimensions to the pharmaceutical industry [6].

The concept of "Quality by Design" has been identified as an approach which has something to do with a developed scientific comprehension of crucial process and product qualities by designing controls and tests on the basis of the scientific limits of comprehension which is determined during the progress, and using the knowledge acquired during the life cycle of the product to improve an amelioration environment permanently in this framework [2].

2.1. ICH Q8

The Q8 guideline is intended to provide guidance on the contents of section 3.2.P.2 (pharmaceutical development) for drug products as defined in module 3 of the common technical document (ICH guideline M4). The pharmaceutical development section aims to provide a comprehensive understanding gained through the application of scientific approaches and quality risk management on the product and the manufacturing process for reviewers and inspectors. The guideline also indicates areas where the greater understanding of pharmaceutical and manufacturing sciences leads to flexible regulatory approaches. The degree of regulatory flexibility is predicated on the level of relevant scientific knowledge provided. It is first produced for the original marketing application and can be updated to support new knowledge gained over the lifecycle of a product [7].

2.2. ICH Q9

QbD is a systematic approach to pharmaceutical development for designing and developing formulations and manufacturing processes that can generate a prescribed product quality. In other words, QbD claims that "quality cannot be tested into products; it should be built-in during the designing phase". Based on this, the ICH guidelines Q9, "quality risk management," and Q10, "pharmaceutical quality system," were published. The guideline Q9 offers principles for quality risk management that can be applied to different aspects of drug quality [1]. The purpose of this document is to offer a systematic approach to quality risk management [8].

Quality risk management tools can be used in various stages of pharmaceutical operations, such as development, production, laboratory controls, packaging, and labeling, and also in inspection and assessment activities. The quality risk management guideline contains two main principles of the risk management model. These principles explain the risk management process and the terminology and tools used for risk evaluation. The aim of the risk management guideline is to create a common understanding to realize risk management, including risks that cover products, processes, and facilities, and risks that affect robustness of the quality system are evaluated, and controls related to risk mitigation are also performed [6].

Consequently, the Q9 explains what risk is, how it is evaluated, and where quality risk management could be applied. It specifically provides guidance on the principles and some quality-risk management tools that can allow making more effective and consistent risk-based decisions by regulators and industry, regarding the quality of drug substances and drug products across the product lifecycle [8].

2.3. ICH Q10

ICH Q10 identifies one multi-purpose model for an effective pharmaceutical quality system which is based on International Standards Organization (ISO) quality concepts and it contains applicable GMP regulations and complements ICH Q8 and ICH Q9. ICH Q10 is a pharmaceutical quality system model that can be implemented throughout different stages of life cycle of a product. Therefore, whether the content of ICH Q10 is additional to the current regional GMP requirements or not is optional. ICH Q10 demonstrates industry and regulatory authorities' support for an effective pharmaceutical quality system to enhance the quality and availability of medicines around the world for public health. Applications of Q10 guideline enables innovation and incessant improvement and empowers the link of pharmaceutical progress. ICH Q10 should be practiced in a way that is appropriate to each product's lifecycle phase [1, 9].

2.4. ICH Q11

ICH Q11, "development and manufacture of the drug substances," was published by ICH in 2012. Q11 was created for drug substances, including biotechnological and biological entities, and is related to drug substance manufacturing and development. Various pharmaceutical development and drug substance understanding approaches are described, and Q11 serves as a guideline on the type of information that should be provided in module 3 CTD sections 3.2.S. 2.2–3.2.S.2.6 [1, 6].

2.5. ICH Q12

ICH Q12, "technical and regulatory considerations for pharmaceutical product life cycle management," is intended to work in compliance with ICH Q8–ICH Q11 guidelines and will give an opportunity to the management of postapproval changes in a more predictable and efficient way throughout the life cycle of the product. After complete pursuance of this guideline, upgraded innovation and continual improvement, and more robust quality assurance and reliable supply of product will be expected. It will allow regulators to better understand, and have more confidence in a firm's pharmaceutical quality system (PQS) for management of post-approval changes [10].

3. QbD road map

QbD is a systematic product development approach that begins with predefined objectives and emphasizes understanding of the product and process based on firm science and quality risk management, as defined in ICH Q8 guideline. Quality risk management and knowledge management are the two basic components of QbD [4].

QbD is a methodical, erudite, risk-oriented, holistic, and proactive approach to pharmaceutical progress that begins with predefined objectives, and underlines product and process comprehension and process control. QbD requires that quality-improving erudite methods might be used upstream in the research, progress, and design phases to ensure that quality is designed into the product process at the earliest possible phase [2].

A vital component of QbD is comprehension of the needs of the patient and the certain quality arrogates of the product concerned to security and impressiveness. Thereby, to apply QbD, it is crucial to have a principal comprehension of the functional relationships among patient necessities, product quality arrogates, analytical abilities, and the production process. QbD works inside the design space (DS) obtained by considering critical formulation and process parameters and so there is no need for product quality verification through final quality test. This knowledge is gained during development and grows with more manufacturing experience through process characterization, scale up, technology transfer, manufacture, and increased patient exposure to the product. This approach makes it feasible to use data gathered from development works performed to create a design space for achieving continuous development. By this way, it is possible to ensure changes in the trade with the change control method, without the need for confirmation from the authority. Regarding the life cycle of the product, the most up-to-date pharmaceutical and engineering information is used [4, 5].

A complete QbD study should include the following four key elements: (i) define a target product quality profile (goals) based on prior scientific knowledge; (ii) design product and manufacturing processes that satisfy predefined goals; (iii) identify potentially high risk attributes and/or parameters and sources of variability by using risk assessment and scientific knowledge to obtain the design space with controlled experimental studies; and (iv) develop a control strategy to control manufacturing processes to produce consistent product quality over time by operating within the established design space, thus assuring that quality is built into the product during the manufacturing, storage, and distribution of the product [2, 11].

Implementation of QbD-based strategies in pharmaceutical development would provide excellence and significant time shortening in product development, and enormous flexibility in regulatory compliance. It has been emphasized before if the principles described in the ICH Q8, Q9, and Q10 guidelines are implemented together in a holistic manner, this will ensure further that the patient will receive product that meets the critical quality attributes (CQAs) [1].

3.1. Determination of quality targets

In order to design quality into a product, the requirements for the product design and performance must be well understood in the early design phase [12]. By beginning with the end in mind, the result of development is a robust formulation and manufacturing process with an acceptable control strategy that ensures the performance of the drug product [11].

Target product profile (TPP) describes the general objective of the pharmaceutical product development program and provides information about the development works. ICH Q8 needs specifying of properties crucial for the quality of the prepared pharmaceutical product, in regard to intended use and route of administration and valuation of intended use of the product and route of administration is performed with the TPP [4]. Pharmaceutical companies will use the desired labeling information to establish a target product profile that describes anticipated indications, contraindications, dosage form, dose, frequency, pharmacokinetics, route of administration, maximum and minimum doses, presentation of pharmaceutical product, and target patient population [12].

The quality target product profile (QTPP) is derived from the desired labeling information for a new product and defined as "a prospective summary of the quality characteristics of a drug product that ideally will be achieved to ensure the desired quality, taking into account safety and efficacy of the drug product" [11, 12]. In addition to defining the design requirements of the product, the QTPP will help identify critical quality attributes such as potency, purity, bioavailability or pharmacokinetic profile, shelf life, and sensory properties [12].

A critical quality attribute is a physical, chemical, biological, or microbiological feature or property that should be within a proper limit, range, or distribution to provide the required product quality [11].

The concept of criticality can be used to explain any feature, importance, or characteristics of an active substance, component, raw material, finished product, or device; or any process characteristics, parameters, conditions, or factors in the finished product [4].

3.2. Determination of critical parameters

A material attribute or process parameter is critical when a realistic change in that attribute or parameter can significantly impact the quality of the output material [11].

The parameter expresses a measurable or countable characteristic of a system or process. Parameters are usually considered as features related to manufacture, such as temperature and mix speed, or as characteristics of equipment or process. Features are considered as characteristics of materials (such as melting point, viscosity, and sterility). However, it must be noted that there are no absolute borders between features and parameters [4].

"Quality attribute hazardousness is initially depended on burden of harm and does not change as a result of exposure management. Process parameter hazardousness is attached to the parameter's effect on any crucial quality arrogates. It is depended on the probability of occurrence and discoverability, so it can change as a result of exposure management" [13].

3.3. Quality risk management

Risk management principles are effectively utilized in many areas of business and government. The importance of quality systems has been affirmed in the pharmaceutical industry too, and it is becoming apparent that quality exposure management is a precious compound of a sufficient quality system.

Commonly, risk is defined as the combination of the probability of occurrence of harm and the severity of that harm. Regarding pharmaceuticals, although there are various stakeholders, including patients and medical practitioners as well as government and industry, the protection of the patient by managing the risk to quality has prime importance.

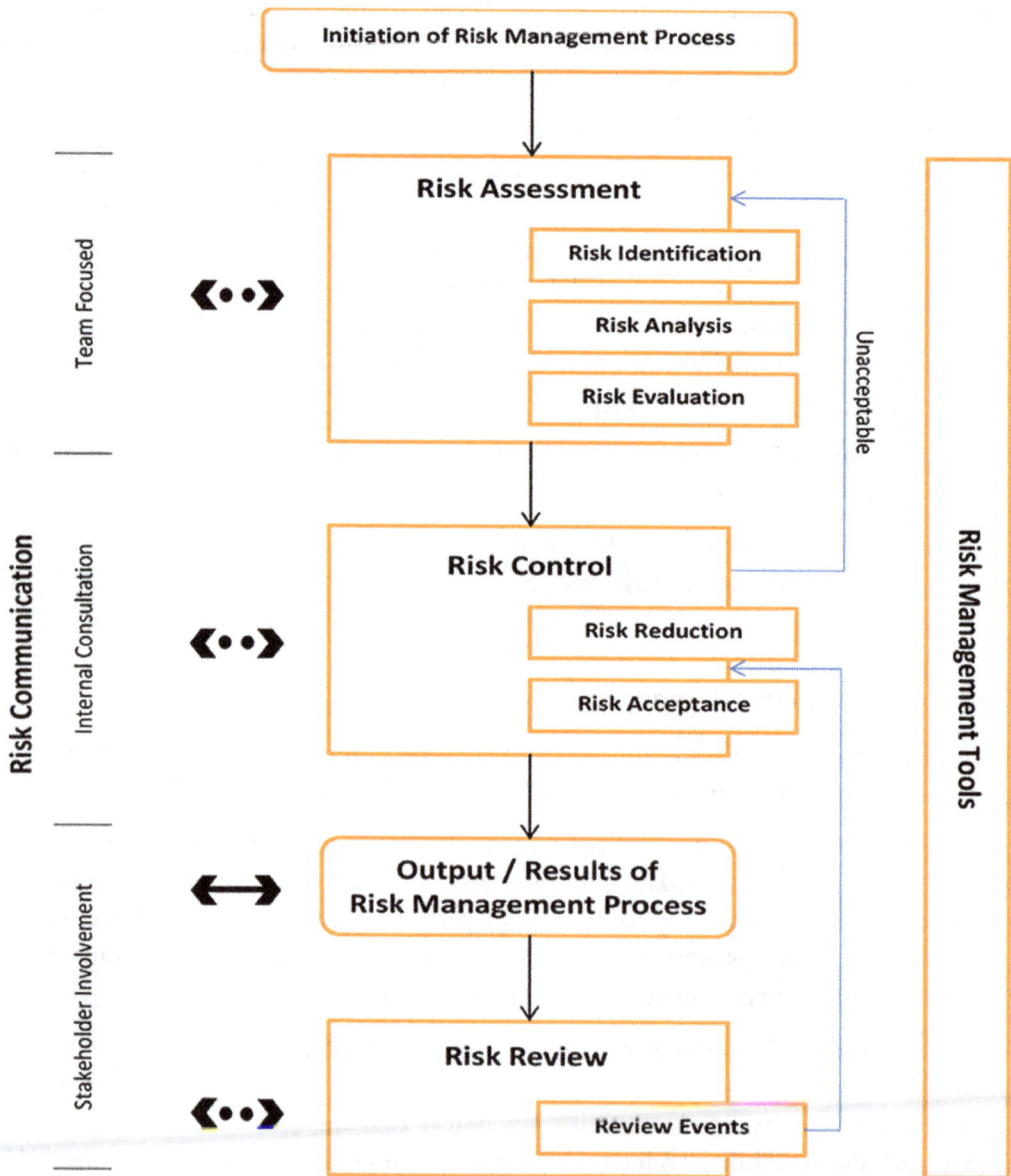

Figure 1. Flow diagram of quality risk management process [8].

ICH Q9 quality risk management provides documented, transparent, and reproducible methods to accomplish quality risk management process steps which are demonstrated in

Figure 1, based on current knowledge about assessing the probability, severity, and sometimes discoverability of the risk. According to the principle, there are two initial principles to consider in quality risk management implementation [8, 11]:

- the valuation of the risk on quality should be dependent on scientific knowledge and accordingly concerned to the protection of the patient; and

- the level of endeavor, circumstance, and documentation of the quality risk management process should be measured with the risk level of the parameter.

Still, traditional approaches like empirical and/ or internal procedures continue to provide useful information on topics such as handling of complaints, quality defects, deviations, and allocation of resources. It has been noted that the pharmaceutical industry and regulators can assess and manage risk using recognized risk management tools and/ or internal procedures (e.g., standard operating procedures). Some of these tools presented in the ICH Q9 guideline are given below:

- Basic risk management facilitation methods like flowcharts;

- Failure mode effects analysis (FMEA);

- Fault tree analysis (FTA);

- Hazard analysis and critical control points (HACCP);

- Risk ranking and filtering; and

- Supporting statistical tools.

It should be proper to comply with these tools for use in certain areas concerned to the medicinal material and the medical product quality. Quality risk management procedures and the adjuvant statistical implements can be utilized in combination. Combined use provides flexibility that can facilitate the implementation of quality risk management principles [8]. According to the guideline, it is important to note that "it is neither always appropriate nor always necessary to use a formal risk management process like recognized tools and/or in-house procedures" [11].

The influential quality risk management approach can further provide the high quality drug (medicinal) product to the patient for ensuring a proactive means to define and control potential quality issues during progress and production. Besides, quality risk management usage can leverage the decision making when a quality matter comes in sight. The influential quality risk management is able to support an erudite and practical approach to decision making [8]. Appropriate use of quality risk management can facilitate but does not obviate industry's obligation to comply with regulatory requirements and does not replace proper communications between industry and regulators [11].

3.3.1. Risk assessment

A well-defined problem description or risk question is the beginning of quality risk assessment. When the risk in question is well defined, an appropriate risk management tool and the types of information needed to address the risk question will be more readily determined. Prior product knowledge is a key in risk assessment and consists of the accumulated laboratory, nonclinical, and clinical experience for any specific product quality attribute. It also can include relevant data from similar molecules and data from literature references. This combined knowledge provides a rationale for relating the attribute to product safety and efficacy [5].

Ishikawa (fishbone) diagram is an effective tool to capture a list of potential process inputs that impacts variation. Mapping the production process using a process flow diagram is beneficial to define the scope of the risk assessment process. FMEA or use of a prioritization matrix is helpful in identifying the process inputs that impact quality attributes [12].

For *Risk identification*, we use the information to identify hazards referring to the risk question or problem. We ask the "What might go wrong?" question, including identifying the possible consequences [8].

Risk analysis is used to estimate of the risk related with the identified hazards by some risk management tools; we can detect the harm with its role in the estimation of risk. Questions such as "What is the likelihood (probability) it will go wrong?", "What are the consequences (severity)?" must be asked to analyze the risk [8].

Risk evaluation compares the identified and analyzed risk against given risk criteria. Risk evaluations consider the strength of evidence for all three of the fundamental questions [8].

3.3.2. Risk control

Risk control decides the level of acceptance of risks which is used for risk control should be proportional to the significance of the risk including benefit-cost analysis, to understand the optimum level of risk control process which might focus on questions below:

- Is the risk above a reasonable level?

- What can be done to diminish or obviate risks?

- What is the proper balance between advantages, risks, and resources?

- Are new risks introduced as a result of the identified risks being controlled?

Risk reduction contains the actions taken to weaken the burden and possibility of harm. The application of risk reduction can introduce new risks into the system.

Risk acceptance can be a decision to accept the residual risk or it can be a decision where residual risks are not specified. For some types of harms, it might be agreed that an appropriate quality risk management strategy has been applied and that quality risk is reduced to an acceptable level [8].

3.3.3. Risk review

Risk management should be a lifelong part of the quality management process. The risk management process should be reviewed to include new knowledge and experience. The frequency of any review should be based on the risk level. Risk review might include reconsideration of risk acceptance decisions [8].

3.3.4. Risk communication

Risk communication is the sharing of information about risk and risk management between the decision makers and others. Parties can communicate at any stage of the risk management process. The outputs of the quality risk management process should be documented. The interested parties might be regulators and industry, industry and the patient, industry or regulatory authority, etc. The information will cover the probability, severity, acceptability, control, treatment, discoverability, or many other aspects of risks to quality [8].

3.4. Design of experiments

While generating design space, parameters to be included or excluded to multiple variation analysis and/or model development should be assessed and selected carefully. There are significant differences between process requirements for large and small molecules, as well as differences between active substance and finished product production phases. When process parameters are defined, number of parameters for multifactorial analysis should be reduced. Generating a design space that includes all parameters that could affect the quality of a product can be long acting and exhausting. Because of this, risk analysis instruments can be used to point at parameters really affecting a CQA in the finished product [14]. Once the CQAs, CPPs, and CMAs are associated with inputs to the process, experiments can be efficiently designed to develop predictive models and confirm causal relationships, through a risk assessment [12].

In recent researches, design of experiments (DoE) has been found as a more efficient system, because it requires less experimental runs, and includes a wider "knowledge space" than traditional changing experimentation with one factor at a time. "Consequently, it is more influential in interrogating conceivable interactions between process factors, avoiding artifacts' such as empirical aggregate and work order with randomization, and making use of "hidden replication," and hereby in having better sensitivity for determining significant effects" [15]. The factors to be studied in a DoE could come from the risk assessment exercise or prior knowledge.

For DoEs with sole or poly unit operations that are used to institute CPPs and/or to define design space, the including of under mentioned information in the submission will extensively assist the valuation by the setters:

- Rationale for selection of DoE variables (including ranges) is risk assessment with alternative or different other instruments. In order to reduce the experiment load necessary for model verification or experiment design, usually it is also possible to divide parameter sets into logical groups. Working on parameters related to single unit operations can allow small groupings be made in product development [14].

- Any evidence of change in raw materials like medicinal material and/or excipients that would have an effect on approximations made from DoE studies.

- Listing of the parameters that would be kept constant during the DoEs and their individual values, consisting of comments on the effect of scale on these parameters.

- Type of empirical current design and a verification of its properness, containing the strength of the design.

- Factors under study and their ranges can be presented in a tabloid format. Supporters should figure out if the factors are abided to be measure-dependent.

- Reference to the type of analytical methods used to evaluate the data and their suitability for their intended use.

- Results and statistical analysis of DoE data showing the statistical significance of the factors and their interactions, including predictions made from DoE studies relevant to scale and equipment differences [13].

3.5. Creating design space

Design space is defined as "multidimensional combinations and interactions of input material variables and process parameters with proven assured quality." Boundaries of the design space should be very well defined. Information should be provided on which parameters and ranges are included in the design space. Comprehensive information about design of experiments and statistical methods should be included in the application [4].

In developing design spaces for existing products, multivariate models can be used for retrospective evaluation of past production data. Design spaces can be based on scientific first principles and/or empirical models. An appropriate statistical design of experiments includes a level of confidence that is valid for the entire design space, including the edges of an approved design space. Additional development knowledge and understanding contributes to design space implementation and continual improvement therefore a design space van be updated over the lifecycle. Risk assessments define the focus of development studies and define the design space as part of the risk management process. Different approaches can be considered when implementing a design space, e.g., process ranges or feedback controls to adjust parameters during processing. The design space associated with the control strategy ensures that the manufacturing process produces product that meets QTPP and CQAs all the time [13].

The design space has been instituted and verified after the process, the regulatory filing would include the reasonable ranges for all key and crucial operating parameters, and a more restricted operating space typically described for drug products. Only movement outside the DS is accepted as change, which typically initiates a regulatory post-approval change process. Activities within the DS are not considered changes [6]. The filing would contain the purified product design space at the same time, definition of the control strategy, outcome of the verification exercise, and plan for process monitoring. The filing could contain procedures in the QbD paradigm at the same time, for instance, comparability protocols or expanded change protocols, which would permit further suppleness in changes concerning preconfirmed criteria that have been complying with between the applicant and the setter [16].

3.6. Control strategy

The control strategy is "a set of planned controls, arising from existing product and process comprehension that warrants process performance and product quality. The controls can contain parameters and attributes, and it is concerned to the medicinal material and drug product materials and components, facility and equipment operating conditions, in-process controls, characterization testing, and the relevant methods and density of observation and audit, comparability tests and stability testing" [11, 15, 16].

The probability of a negative impact on product safety and efficacy can be minimized by a holistic approach to the control strategy. The aim of a control strategy for a product is to provide that influential controls are in place to pursue the risks connected with the product at a tolerable level. Therefore, the understandings of risk management and control strategy are profoundly associated and the use of risk assessment in creating the control strategy is unique to the QbD approach [16]. The control strategy creates layers of protection that reduce the risk of the hazards creating actual harm [15]. Additional emphasis on process controls should be considered in cases where products cannot be well-characterized and/or quality attributes might not be readily measurable due to limitations of testing or discoverability.

When designing the control strategy, the identification and linkage of the CQAs and CPPs should be considered. A well-developed control strategy will reduce risk but does not change the criticality of attributes. The control strategy plays a key role in ensuring that the CQAs are met, and hence that the QTPP is realized [13]. A well-designed control strategy that results from appropriate leveraging of Q8/Q9/Q10 principles leads to reliable product quality and patient-safety profiles. Design space boundaries are an integral part of a comprehensive control strategy. The control strategy for a product is expected to evolve through the product lifecycle. As product knowledge evolves and changes including acceptance criteria, analytical methodology, or the points of control (e.g., introduction of real-time release testing), there is the possibility of less reliance on end-product testing [15]. The permanent process validation is an approach which permits a firm for observing the process and make amendments to the process and/or the control strategy correspondingly. If multivariate prediction models are used in systems that pursue and update the models help to warrant the permanent convenience of the model within the control strategy [16].

3.7. Process analytical technology

There is a shift from lab-based end-product quality testing to better formulation and process design, leading potentially to more in-line, online or at-line testing.

Process analytical technology (PAT) is defined as a system for analyzing and controlling manufacturing through timely measurements of critical quality and performance attributes of raw and in-process materials and processes during the processes. This is for the goal of ensuring final product quality. The goal of PAT is to support principles of QbD that emphasize fundamental process understanding and control focus to maximize process efficiency. The main PAT tools can be divided into two main groups as multivariate data acquisition and analysis and modern process analyzers or process analytical chemistry tools [17].

3.8. Continual improvement

Continuous improvement is an essential factor in a modern quality system that aims developing efficiency by leveraging a process and removing wasted endeavors in production. These endeavors are being initially directed toward in order to diminish variability in process and product quality attributions.

The pharmaceutical quality system has to enable permanent development and assist to describe and implement proper product quality developments, process developments, changefulness diminution, innovations, and quality system enhancements, thus increasing the capability to fulfill quality necessities permanently. Quality risk management can be helpful for describing and prioritizing points for permanent development.

Examples of continuous improvement include actions like adjusting a set point of a process, advanced control techniques, redesigning a process step, simplifying documents, installing online measurements, changing the design space and updating the control strategy data for continuous improvement [18].

3.9. Benefits and challenges of the QbD implementation

There are of course some challenges in implementing the QbD approach like *training*, which is a major challenge; therefore, regulatory authorities and industry should conduct the training program for the implementation of the QbD concept.

It is relatively a new concept to the pharmaceutical industry and there is still a *lack of understanding and trust* among all parties so it is important to share proprietary information with especially regulatory groups.

Associated costs to implement QbD in product development, manufacturing unit operations (business and marketing decisions), different regulatory processes (BLA, NDA, ANDA, follow-on, and so on), and associated regulatory practices and culture are current concerns and establishing balance between QbD-based versus traditional demonstration of quality is in transition [17].

However, gains in the process make the implementation of the QbD indispensable. The benefits of QbD span the product lifecycle and center on areas that have the most impact to the safety, efficacy, and quality of the product and encourage innovation and continuous improvement to the product long after initial approval to leverage knowledge gained and technology advancements [3]. From the perspective of manufacturers, better understanding of product/process, development of more effective processes and less regulatory requirements are possible. In addition to these, it permits for concepts crucial and noncrucial parameters in improving design space, ensures the opportunity for centering upon significant parameters of product quality in verification works [4].

QbD provides potential opportunities for real-time quality control and reduction of the end point (QC) release testing; decreased final product testing and lower batch release costs, reduced batch failure rates; so lower operating costs from fewer failures and deviation investigations; also reduced raw material and finished product inventory costs; ensures better design of the products with fewer problems in manufacturing; allows for the implementation of new technology to improve manufacturing without regulatory scrutiny; and ensures less complication during review, so that reduced deficiencies and quicker approval is possible [17].

Another benefit often noted is the promise of less burdensome regulatory reporting of postapproval changes. Even without the incentive of less burdensome regulatory oversight [3].

4. Quality by design approach for biotechnology products

As in past few decades, manufacturers define a process and aim to perform the process consistently in a way that the critical parameters are controlled within a narrow range in order to reduce versatility in product quality for biotechnology products. However, because the process controls are fixed in this approach, any variability in raw materials, environmental controls, and/or process operations manifests as variability in product quality and results in lot failures [19]. The international ICH Q8 (R2), Q9, and Q10 guidelines provide the foundation for implementing QbD to the biotech products, however, involve some differences and complexities [5].

A key element in implementing QbD for biotechnology products is engineering the molecule itself. A number of strategies are currently used by investigators to alter the properties of the molecule to achieve the desired balance among efficacy, stability, safety, and manufacturability. Realization of the structure and functional attributes of therapeutic proteins, including monoclonal antibodies (MAbs), is crucial to create the design space, because that understanding facilitates the selection of requested quality attributes through the molecular design while ensuring that bioactivity of the protein therapeutic is maintained [5].

There is a need for certain technologies and processes for QbD implementation in the biopharmaceutical industry. Extensive data about the product and its manufacturing process is required for QbD implementation. It is not possible to evaluate the effect of every variable numerous variables and attributes that show interaction to impact safety and efficacy of a biotechnology product. Statistical approaches, such as DOE and multivariate data analysis (MVDA) along with risk management tools, can help to ensure that resources are spent on the most important tasks [19]. Currently, authorities have not submitted the clear guidance on what they take into consideration to be a reasonable risk for biotechnology products. The industry is able to work with health authorities for sharing examples of process changes and to ensure an evaluation for postapproval variations and notification categorization. There is no clearly defined mechanism to share process understanding for well-understood processes and products [3].

According to information given above, basic QbD approaches for biotechnological products and their manufacturing are QTPP and CQAs. Because of unique nature of the bioproducts/bioprocesses, multivariate QTTP parameters are at stake. For this reason, QbD approaches for monoclonal antibodies will be considered in the chapter.

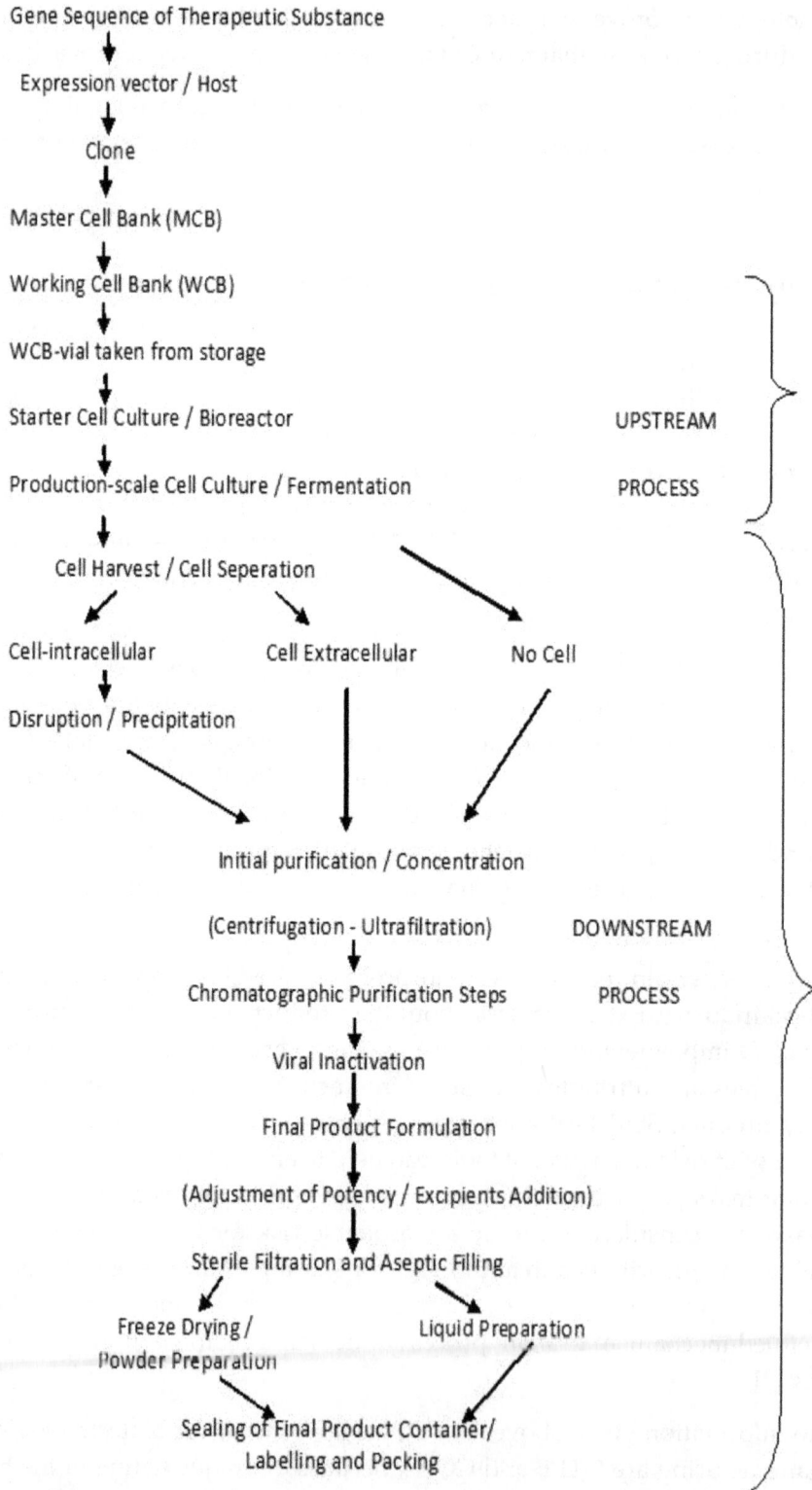

Figure 2. Standard production process flow diagram (biotechnological products) [20–22].

In **Figure 2**, basic bioprocessing steps are given for better understanding of QTTP and CQAs for biotechnological products. In the downstream process, various purification methods are integrated as seen. Selection of one of the chromatographic methods given in **Table 1** depends on the drug substance characteristics, cell line and bioreactor choices, and other process-related properties.

Chromatographic method	Principle
Size-exclusion (Gel-filtration) chromatography	Size/shape difference
Ion-exchange chromatography	Net surface charge difference, pH
Affinity chromatography	Biological affinity between drug substance and ligand (metal chelates, lectins, dyes)
Hydrophobic interaction chromatography	Surface hydrophobicity difference, polarity
Immunoaffinity	Purification of Mab, based on affinity between Mab and antigen (protein A, protein G)
Hydroxyapatite chromatography	Complex interaction between drug substance and media
İmmobilized metal-ion affinity	Metal-ion binding
Chromatofocusing	Isoelectric point difference

Source: [20, 22, 24, 26].

Table 1. Types of chromatographic methods used in downstream process of biotech products.

In downstream processing of Mabs, purification steps are similar to the other biotech products but also contain specific methods such as protein A chromatography which is commonly used for its IgG (Mab) affinity. This method distinguishes itself by high selectivity toward IgG-type antibodies, high flow rate, and capacity [20, 23–25].

In large-scale production of biopharmaceuticals, there are optimization criteria for bioprocess development; concentration, volumetric productivity, yield (high titer), and quality (sequence, purity, glycosylation pattern, activity). Optimization begins with identification and characterization of the drug molecule as well as its mode of action. In the light of this information; cell culture processing (cell engineering, production cell line selection, type of bioreactor and critical parameters, feeding strategy (batch, fed-batch, perfusion, continuous), downstream process steps and parameters, process monitoring, analytics and formulation studies) is designed in compliance with regulatory requirements [22, 24, 27, 28].

In terms of identification and characterization, monoclonal antibodies (Mabs) can be considered as an example for drug-substance properties. Mabs are produced by hybridoma technology and its basic concept is producing identical antibodies and simply includes these steps [20, 29]:

Critical process attributes   Critical process parameters

Viability   Working Cell Bank (WCB)   Temperature
Cell counting   ↓   Time
                                 WCB- vial taken from storage

Product viability   ↓   Temperature
Culture viability   Starter Cell Culture / Bioreactor   Culture duration
Cell density / Biomass   Agitation
Ph,   +   Gas flow rate
dO$_2$, dCO$_2$ Shear forces
Aggregate   Bubble size distribution
Primary structure   Osmolality
Post-translational profile   Production-scale Cell Culture / Fermentation   Anti-foam concentration
                                                                                Feed-batch composition,
                                                                                volume and timing
                                                                                Glycosilation pattern
                                                                                Deamidated isoforms

Product yield   Cell Harvest / Cell Seperation
Viability at harvest
Cell debris   Pressure
Biomass   Cell-intracellular   Cell Extracellular   No Cell   Flow rate
                                                                                Temperature

Product yield   Homogenization / Precipitation   pH, Pressure
Viability   (Cell disruption)   Conductivity (supernate)

Product yield   pH
Viability   Initial purification / Concentration   G-force
Turbidity   Duration of centrifugation
Filter integrity   (Centrifugation - Ultrafiltration)   Nonviable cell density
                                            ↓   Particle size distribution

Highly purified product   Protein load
Bioburden reduction   Protein A Chrom.   Elution Buffer pH
Endotoxin   ↓

Adventitious virus   Time
Aggregate   Viral Inactivation   Temperature
Charge variants   (Low pH)   Ph
                                            ↓

Host cell protein (HCP)   Load/wash conductivity
Residual DNA   Ion-Exchange Chrom.   Elution buffer pH
Bioburden/endotoxin   Flow rate
Aggregate   (Anion/Cation)

Adventitious virus   ↓   Filtration volume
Aggregate   Small Virus filtration   Pressure
Filter integrity   Integrity test
                                            ↓

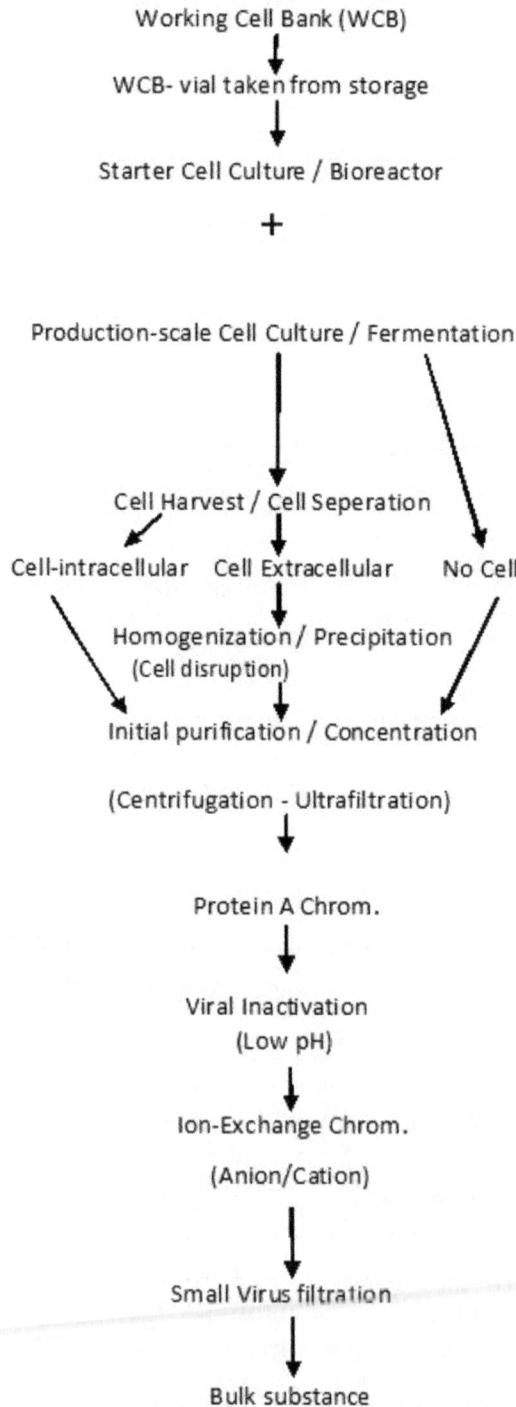

                                      Bulk substance

Figure 3. Control strategy for upstream and downstream processes of biomanufacturing. dO$_2$: dissolved oxygen, dCO$_2$: dissolved carbon dioxide [22–27, 30–34].

<u>Critical process attributes</u>

Identity
Potency
Charge Heterogeniety
Quantity / Titer
Particulate matter
Purity/impurities
Clarity
Sterility

Bulk substance

(Adjustment of Potency)

<u>Critical process parameters</u>

Molecular integrity
Isoform pattern
Glycosylation profile
Electrophoretic pattern
Chromatographic pattern
Spectroscopic profiles
Acidic/basic variants
Protein content/ Biomass
Molecular weight
Aggregates
Bioburden/endotoxin
Adventitious virus
Host Cell Protein (HCP)

Drug substance
concentration
Excipient concentration
Raw material impurities
Particulate matter
Container
Biocompability
Ph
Aggregation
Oxidation
Bioburden

Formulation

(Addition of Excipients / Compounding)

Protein content/ Biomass
Aggregates
Glycosylation pattern
pH adjustment
Visible/subvisible particles
HCP
Compounding mixing time, mixing speed, hold time
Temperature

Filter integrity
Pressure
Aggregation
Oxidation
Bioburden/endotoxin
Particulate matter
Sterility
Vial filling rate
Fill-line operation

Sterile Filtration and

Aseptic Filling

Filter size
Flow rate, Flushing volume
integrity test
Holding time
Aggregate
Bioburden reduction
Particulate Removal
Homogeniety
Filler speed, pressure

Dosage form
Protein content per vial
pH
Reconstitution Time
Cryoprotectants
Stabilizing excipients

Freeze Drying / Powder Preparation   **Liquid Preparation**

Ph adjustment
Aggregation
Denaturation
Crystallization

Biopotency
Dose
Mode of administration
Charge Heterogeniety
Post-translational profile
Osmolality
Color
Sterility
Shelf life
Storage temperature
Container
Biocompatibility
Purity / impurities
Pharmacopoeial compliance
Particulate matter

Final Product

(Sealing of Final Product Container/

Labelling and Packing)

Sequence mutation
Truncated antibodies
Molecular integrity
Isoform pattern
Glycosylation profile
Electrophoretic pattern
Chromatographic pattern
Spectroscopic profiles
Acidic/basic variants
Protein content/ Biomass
Aggregate
Conductivity
Mass balance
Visible/subvisible particles
Duration of time at
specified temperature

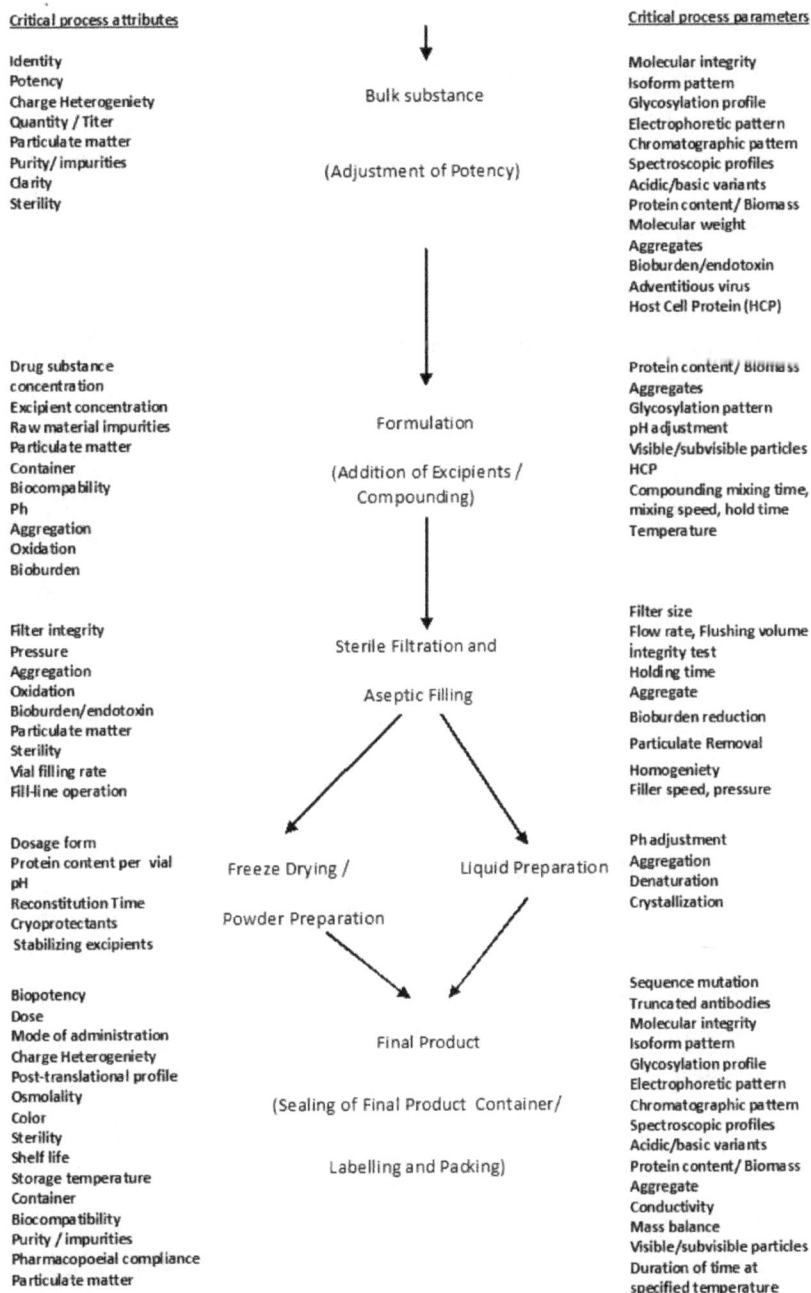

Figure 4. Control strategy for drug substance and final product processes [22–27, 30–34].

- immunization of mouse with antigen

- isolation of B cells (contains antibodies)

- cell fusion with myeloma cells (immortal B cell cancer cells)

- screening and selection of hybrids and propagation

- selecting positive clones, freezing the clones

- production of ascites and harvest specific antibody

Mabs consist of constant Fc regions and constant/variable Fab regions. Fc regions have heavy chains, while Fab regions have both heavy and light chains. The Fc region is responsible for biological activity. Variable light chains (VL) of the Fab region are responsible for antigen recognition and binding. There are four types of Mabs used for therapy; murine, chimeric, humanized, and human Mabs. Murine Mabs consist of overall murine amino acids, while chimeric Mabs' only variable regions are murine originated, humanized Mabs' complementarity determining regions (CDRs) are murine originated, and human IgG consists of entirely human amino acids [29].

Humanized and human Mabs are preferred for their reduced risk of heterogeneity and negative impact on bioactivity. Determination of critical attributes and parameters for Mab products depends on overall structure of Mab, cell clone, and media. Complementarity determining regions (CDRs) of the heavy and light chains have potential glycosylation, deamidation, and oxidation sites, which pose risks such as undesirable glycosylation profiles, disulphide bond formation, and oxidation [29].

Product heterogeneity is a common problem for all recombinant biotechnological products as well as for Mabs. This could occur either in cell culture process or downstream process and eliminating these variants all along manufacturing process is one of basic approaches of QbD. These variants such as aggregates, deamidation and oxidation products, and different glycosylation patterns strongly affect product's quality, potency, bioavailability, and immunogenicity which could be fatal. In **Figures 3** and **4**, key process attributes and related critical parameters are outlined in parallel with biomanufacturing steps and further information is given within the article [29].

Cell line, bioreactor, and medium selection and design are based on cell culture process approaches. Control strategies of pH, oxygen (O_2), carbon dioxide (CO_2), temperature, and pressure are determinant for optimization and scaleup [27]:

- pH control strategy; basically based on correlation between CO_2 addition and base addition which is related to osmolality, pH, and CO_2.

- O_2 control strategy; depends on agitation, gas flow rate, and orifice diameter which is related to dO_2, dCO_2, shear forces, mixing, and bubble-size distribution.

- temperature control strategy; based on temperature, which is related to O_2 and CO_2 solubilities.

- pressure control strategy; based on pressure, which is related to O_2 and CO_2 solubilities.

According to these attributes, physical parameters such as gas flow rate, agitation speed, shear stress; chemical parameters such as dO_2, dCO_2, pH, osmolality, and by-product and substrate metabolites and biological parameters such as cell viability and concentration are critical parameters for the cell culture process. Even minor variations in these parameters could have very strong impact on productivity, product quality, and potency. Thus, these parameters must be characterized and optimized. Some of these parameters are measured by direct connection to the operator but some need to be measured via intervention. For example, viability is measured through cell counting tests such as hemocytometer [27].

Before selecting the cell line, small scale production of chosen cells (*Escherichia coli*, yeast, insect cell, mammalian cells) are carried out and the cell with best performance in terms of activity, speed, and solubility is selected for large-scale production. Post-translational processing and stable expression are critical parameters for selection. For example, mammalian cells (CHO, mouse myeloma cells) have closer glycosylation pattern to human and ensure stable expression, thus these cells are commonly used for Mab production [24, 27, 35].

Bioreactor and culture media selection and design approaches should meet defined product quality, productivity, and cell-line specifications. Bioreactor is operated by batch, fed-batch, or continuous modes and the choice of bioreactor based on two criteria; productivity and sterility. Continuous systems ensure high productivity but cleaning is a matter of fact. Disposable bioreactor systems seem to be a good alternative for production; however, they need to be optimized. Critical parameters for design strategy are; reactor type, mixing, temperature, density, shear stress, gas exchange (O_2-CO_2), perfusion rate, and ease of cleaning [24, 27].

Commonly used cell culture medium supplements consist of glucose, amino acids, inorganic salts, vitamins, growth factors, and animal component free hydrolysates. However, medium ingredients vary due to the high diversity of cell culture properties and medium optimization becomes compulsory for optimal growth of the culture [24, 27].

Basic approaches of the feeding strategy are; maintaining culture viability, promoting growth, increasing productivity and cell density, cost, and time-effectiveness for industrial-scale production. This requires optimization of feed composition in a timely manner and balancing between nutrient consumption and by-product accumulation (ammonium lactate) which is specific for individual cell lines. Combination systems with high-throughput screening and/or statistical design of experiment (DOE) approaches provide ideal formulations for achieving the maximum cell growth and volumetric productivity. Using anti-apoptotic molecules is another approach for prolonging cell viability to increase productivity [24, 27, 36, 37].

Optimization approaches in downstream processing (DSP) are; yield, purity, productivity, larger process capabilities, and faster process development. DSP based on various filtration and chromatographic operation units, which consist of viral-inactivation and final sterile filtration steps. Removal of contaminants and impurities such as residual cell, media components, host cell protein (HCP), residual DNA, product variants, adventitious viruses, endotoxin, aggregates, and other process related impurities is very crucial for producing products suitable for human use. Among other impurities; product variants, aggregates, and host cell protein (HCP) are most important in activity, efficacy, or safety aspects. First purification step is recovery of the drug substance from cell culture and removal of cell/cell debris, fluid. This process is operated by centrifugation/ultrafiltration and if needed microfiltration steps. These steps are determinant for success of further purification process. Chromatographic steps are critical for high degree of purity and recovery. Design of ligands/matrices of chromatographic methods should be optimized for shorter residence time, higher flow rates, and longer lifecycles, which results in increased binding capacity and improved removal of impurities in washing steps. Primary critical parameters for optimization are; viability, yield, aggregates, isoforms, HCP, residual DNA, and turbidity. Most of the overall manufacturing costs derive from downstream processing and increase in parallel with higher yield. The main approach for integrating purification steps is increasing titer with cost-cutting measures. Process development is achieved by PAT-QbD systems, high-throughput screening, continuous processing, small-scale/parallel facilities, and integration of modeling [22, 24–26, 30, 31, 34].

Quality attribute	Analytical assay	Quality assessment criteria
Molecule integrity/ weight	PM/MS, cDNA sequence, IEF, CE-SDS or SDS-PAGE	Amino acid sequence/antibody mutation
Biopotency	Immunoassay, biological activity tests	Target antigen binding affinity
Color, clarity	Colorless, clear	
Aggregation/fragments	HP-SEC, electrophoresis	High levels of aggregation, risk of immunogenicity
Glycosylation	HPLC or CE based glycan assay	High levels of different glycosylation forms
Charge heterogeneity	IEF, ion exchange chromatography, or HPLC	High levels of acidic or basic variant/peaks
Process-related impurities	Immunoassay, DNA-hybridization, Q-PCR, electron microscopy, *in vivo/in vitro* assays, spectral analysis	Avoid HCP, leached Protein A, DNA, viruses, cell culture medium proteins
Particulate matter	Visible/sub-visible particles USP	Meet USP 788 requirements
Bioburden/endotoxin	LAL test	Meet USP 85 requirements
Thermal stability	DSC	According to specified temperature

CE, capillary electrophoresis; IEF, isoelectric focusing; SDS-PAGE, sodium dodecyl sulphate polyacrylamide gel electrophoresis; HP-SEC, high-pressure size exclusion chromatography; PM/MS, peptide mapping-mass spectrometry; DSC, differential scanning calorimetry. *Source*: [25, 27, 28, 30, 31, 38].

Table 2. Drug product specifications in biotechnological manufacturing.

Drug product quality attributes and criteria are given in **Table 2** and the main goal of the QbD design is to match these criteria and guarantee defined quality for drug product at the end of the manufacturing process. At this point, process monitoring by biosensors is very critical throughout manufacturing. Especially monitoring of biomass and cell volumes is the most important. Primary physical, chemical, and biological parameters monitored by sensors are genetic/metabolic analysis, biomass/viability, product characteristics, product concentration, impurities, temperature, osmolality, nutrients, metabolites/substrates, pH, dissolved O_2, volume/weight, CO_2 rate, flow pressure, stirrer speed, viscosity, and side components. Also, biosensors should match some criteria in order to be valid for quality assurance; such as robustness, reliability, accuracy, reproducibility, analysis frequency, selectivity, sensitivity, linearity, ease of cleaning, and sterility [26, 28, 35].

Author details

Buket Aksu[1], Ali Demir Sezer[2*], Gizem Yeğen[1] and Lale Kusçu[2]

*Address all correspondence to: adsezer@marmara.edu.lı

1 Faculty of Pharmacy, Pharmaceutical Technology Department, Istanbul Kemerburgaz University, Bakırköy, Istanbul, Turkey

2 Faculty of Pharmacy, Pharmaceutical Biotechnology Department, Marmara University, Haydarpasa, Istanbul, Turkey

References

[1] Aksu B., Paradkar A., Matas M., Özer Ö., Güneri T., York P. Quality by Design Approach: Application of Artificial Intelligence Techniques of Tablets Manufactured by Direct Compression. AAPS PharmSciTech, 2012; 13(4): 1138–1146.

[2] Aksu B., Paradkar A., Matas M., Özer Ö., Güneri T., York P. A quality by Design Approach Using Artificial Intelligence Techniques to Control the Critical Quality Attributes of Ramipril Tablets Manufactured by Wet Granulation. Pharm Dev Technol, 2013; 18(1): 236–245.

[3] Rathore A.S., et. al. Quality by Design for Biotechnology Products - Part 3. Biopharm Int, 2010; 23(1): 36–45.

[4] Aksu B. Quality by Design (QbD) Roadmap. Control Released Society Indian Chapter, 2015; 7: 25–28.

[5] Arora T., et. al. Quality by Design for Biotechnology Products - Part 1. Biopharm Int, 2009; 22(11): 26–36.

[6] Aksu B., Aydoğan M., Kanık B., Aksoy E. A Flexible Regulatory Approach for Different Raw Materials Suppliers Using QbD Principles. Res J Pharm Biol Chem Scie (RJPBCS), 2013; 4(4): 358–372.

[7] Pharmaceutical Development Q8(R2), ICH Harmonised Tripartite Guideline, 2009.

[8] Quality Risk Management Q9, ICH Harmonised Tripartite Guideline, 2005.

[9] Pharmaceutical Quality System Q10, ICH Harmonised Tripartite Guideline, 2008.

[10] Final Concept Paper Q12: Technical and Regulatory Considerations for Pharmaceutical Product Lifecycle Management. International Conference on Harmonisation of Technical Requirements for Registration of Pharmaceuticals for Human Use (ICH), (Endorsed) 2014.

[11] Pharmaceutical Development Report Example QbD for MR Generic Drugs. Quality by Design for ANDAs: An Example for Modified Release Dosage Forms, 2011.

[12] McCurdy V. Quality by Design in Process Understanding: For Scale-Up and Manufacture of Active Ingredients, 1st ed. Edited by Ian Houson,Wiley-VCH, Germany, 2011.

[13] ICH Quality Implementation Working Group Points to Consider (R2), ICH-Endorsed Guide for ICH Q8/Q9/Q10 Implementation, International Conference on Harmonisation of Technical Requirements for Registration of Pharmaceuticals for Human Use (ICH), 2011.

[14] Aksu B., Yegen G. New Quality Concepts in Pharmaceuticals. MÜSBED, 2014; 4(2): 96–104.

[15] Rathore A.S., et. al. Quality by Design for Biotechnology Products—Part 2. Biopharm Int, 2009; 22(12): 42–58.

[16] Roy S. Quality by Design: A Holistic Concept of Building Quality in Pharmaceuticals. Int J Pharm Biomed Res, 2012; 3(2): 100–108.

[17] Varu R. K., Khanna A. Opportunities and Challenges to Implementing Quality by Design Approach in Generic Drug Development. J Gen Med, 2010; 7: 60–73.

[18] Trivedi B, et al. Quality by Design (QbD) in Pharmaceuticals. Int J Pharm Pharm Sci, 2012; 4(1): 17–29.

[19] Rathore A.S. Quality by Design for Biologics and Biosimilars. PharmTechnol. 2011; 35(3): 64–68.

[20] Walsh G, editor. Pharmaceutical Biotechnology — Concepts and Applications. John Wiley & Sons Ltd. West Sussex, England. 2007. 121–171.

[21] Conner J.,Wuchterl D., Lopez M., Minshall B., Prusti R., Boclair D., Peterson J., Allen. Chapter 26; The Biomanufacturing of Biotechnology Products. In: Craig Shimasaki, editor. Biotechnology Entrepreneurship. 1st ed. Elsevier, Inc., Oxford, UK. 2014; 351–385.

[22] Sommerfeld S., Strube J. Challenges in biotechnology production—Generic Processes and Process Optimization for Monoclonal Antibodies. Chem Eng Process. 2005; 44(10): 1123–1137.

[23] Arora I. Chromatographic Methods for the Purification of Monoclonal Antibodies and Their Alternatives: A Review. Int J Emer Technol and Adv Eng. 2013; 3(10): 475–481.

[24] Gronemeyer P., Ditz R., Strube J. Trends in Upstream and Downstream Process Development for Antibody Manufacturing. Bioengineering J Review, 2014; 1: 188–212.

[25] Liu H.F., Ma J., Winter C., Bayer R. Recovery and Purification Process Development for Monoclonal Antibody Production. Mabs J. 2010; 2(5): 480–499.

[26] Meitz A., Sagmeister P., Langemann T., Herwig C. An Integrated Downstream Process Development Strategy Along QbD Principles. Bioengineering J. 2014; 1(4): 213–230.

[27] Li F., Vijayasankaran N., Shen A.Y., Kiss R., Amanullah A. Cell Culture Processes for Monoclonal Antibody Production. Mabs J. 2010, 2(5): 466–477.

[28] Pohlscheidt M.,Charaniya S., Bork C., Jenzsch M., Noetzel T.L., Luebbert A. Chapter 69; Bioprocess and Fermentation Monitoring. In: Michael C. Flickinger, editor. Upstream Industrial Biotechnology: Equipment, Process Design, Sensing, Control, and cGMP Operations, Volume 2, 1st ed. John Wiley & Sons, Inc., New York, USA. 2013; 2: 1471–1491.

[29] Weiner G.J. Building Better Monoclonal Antibody-Based Therapeutics. Nature Reviews Cancer. Macmillan Publishers Ltd. 2015; 15: 361–370.

[30] A-Mab: A Case Study in Bioprocess Development. Product Development and Realisation Case Study A-Mab. CMC Biotech Working Group, Version2.1. Bangkok, Tailand. 2009; 25–278.

[31] Feroz J.F.,Hershenson S., Khan M.A., Martin-Moe S., editors. Quality by Design for Biopharmaceutical Drug Product Development. Springer, LLC. New York, USA. 2015. 1–86, 117–190, 511–536.

[32] FDA Guidance for Industry: Q8(R2) Pharmaceutical Development. Revision 2, 2009.

[33] ICH Harmonised Tripartite Guideline Q6B. Specifications: Test Procedures and Acceptance Criteria for Biotechnological / Biological Products, Current Step 4 Version, 1999.

[34] Rathore A.S. Roadmap for Implementation of Quality by Design (QbD) for Biotechnology Products. Trends in Biotechnology, 2009; 27(9): 546–553.

[35] Optimization for Monoclonal Antibodies. Chemical Engineering and Processing: Process Intensification, 2005; 44(10): 1123–1137.

[36] Kuchibhatla J., Hunt C., Holdread S., Brooks J.W. A Rapid and Effective Screening Process of Animal Component Free Hydrolysates to Increase Cell Performance. In: IBC Bioprocess International Conference, LR876. 4–7 October 2004; Boston, MA.

[37] Fletcher T. Designing Culture Media for Recombinant Protein Production a Rational Approach. Bioprocess Int, 2005; 3: 30–36.

[38] Sushila D. Chavan S.D, Pimpodkar N.V., Kadam A.S, Gaikwad P.S. Quality by Design. Research and Reviews: J Pharm Qual Assur (JPQA), 2015; 1(2): 18–24.

Permissions

The contributors of this book come from diverse backgrounds, making this book a truly international effort. This book will bring forth new frontiers with its revolutionizing research information and detailed analysis of the nascent developments around the world.

We would like to thank all the contributing authors for lending their expertise to make the book truly unique. They have played a crucial role in the development of this book. Without their invaluable contributions this book wouldn't have been possible. They have made vital efforts to compile up to date information on the varied aspects of this subject to make this book a valuable addition to the collection of many professionals and students.

This book was conceptualized with the vision of imparting up-to-date information and advanced data in this field. To ensure the same, a matchless editorial board was set up. Every individual on the board went through rigorous rounds of assessment to prove their worth. After which they invested a large part of their time researching and compiling the most relevant data for our readers.

The editorial board has been involved in producing this book since its inception. They have spent rigorous hours researching and exploring the diverse topics which have resulted in the successful publishing of this book. They have passed on their knowledge of decades through this book. To expedite this challenging task, the publisher supported the team at every step. A small team of assistant editors was also appointed to further simplify the editing procedure and attain best results for the readers.

Apart from the editorial board, the designing team has also invested a significant amount of their time in understanding the subject and creating the most relevant covers. They scrutinized every image to scout for the most suitable representation of the subject and create an appropriate cover for the book.

The publishing team has been an ardent support to the editorial, designing and production team. Their endless efforts to recruit the best for this project, has resulted in the accomplishment of this book. They are a veteran in the field of academics and their pool of knowledge is as vast as their experience in printing. Their expertise and guidance has proved useful at every step. Their uncompromising quality standards have made this book an exceptional effort. Their encouragement from time to time has been an inspiration for everyone.

The publisher and the editorial board hope that this book will prove to be a valuable piece of knowledge for researchers, students, practitioners and scholars across the globe.

List of Contributors

John J. Bowling, William R. Shadrick and Elizabeth C. Griffith
Department of Chemical Biology and Therapeutics, St. Jude Children's Research Hospital, Memphis, TN, United States

Richard E. Lee
Department of Chemical Biology and Therapeutics, St. Jude Children's Research Hospital, Memphis, TN, United States
Department of Pharmaceutical Sciences, University of Tennessee Health Science Center, Memphis, TN, United States

Yu-Chen Lo
Department of Bioengineering, Stanford University, Stanford, CA, USA

Jorge Z. Torres
Department of Chemistry and Biochemistry, University of California, Los Angeles, CA, USA

Tingting Xu and Steven Ripp
Center for Environmental Biotechnology, The University of Tennessee, Knoxville, USA

Michael Conway, Ashley Frank, Amelia Brumbaugh and Dan Close
BioTech, Knoxville, Tennessee, USA

Josse R. Thomas
Faculty of Pharmaceutical Sciences, KU Leuven, Leuven, Belgium

Chris van Schravendijk
Faculty of Medicine and Pharmacy, Vrije Universiteit Brussel, Brussels, Belgium

Lucia Smit
Braingain, Empowering Young Professionals, Brussels, Belgium

Luciano Saso
Faculty of Pharmacy and Medicine, Sapienza University of Rome, Rome, Italy

Naiara Clemente Tavares, Pedro Henrique Nascimento de Aguiar, Sandra Grossi Gava and Marina Moraes Mourão
Rene Rachou Research Center, FIOCRUZ, Belo Horizonte, Minas Gerais, Brazil

Guilherme Oliveira
Vale Institute of Technology – ITV, Belém, Pará, Brazil

Shane R. Horman
Advanced Assays, Genomics Institute of the Novartis Research Foundation, San Diego, CA, USA

Buket Aksu and Gizem Yeğen
Faculty of Pharmacy, Pharmaceutical Technology Department, Istanbul Kemerburgaz University, Bakırköy, Istanbul, Turkey

Ali Demir Sezer and Lale Kusçu
Faculty of Pharmacy, Pharmaceutical Biotechnology Department, Marmara University, Haydarpasa, Istanbul, Turkey

Index

www.ingramcontent.com/pod-product-compliance
Lightning Source LLC
Chambersburg PA
CBHW062006190326
41458CB00009B/2984

* 9 7 8 1 6 3 2 4 2 5 8 6 7 *